Preface

'Surgery is a branch of human biology that occasionally requires a dissection under anaesthesia.' (Anonymous)

'Swan in, mind off.' (Anonymous)

'... where is the machine that goes PING?' (*Monty Python's the Meaning of Life*)

This book is directed towards those individuals who are involved in the intensive care management of cardiothoracic patients. It is designed to be used not only as a self-assessment review for those preparing for certifying examinations, but also to provide a reference for both common and uncommon problems. Thus, the bulk of the scenarios and discussion are designed for house officers, residents, fellows and registrars. Recognizing that there are individuals from different specialties involved, and that certifying examinations vary between specialties as well as between countries, the questions and answers are designed to reflect different examinations. Some are written so as to prime an individual for an oral examination, some for multiple choice and some for written essay-type examinations. Finally, these questions are also designed to be used as a teaching tool for more junior medical professionals and, in particular, medical students. It is the authors' hope that the questions might be used to illustrate teaching points. For instance, it is not uncommon during an oral cardiac examination for a student to be asked to draw out valvular anatomy and discuss aspects of surgical management. To illustrate this, we have deliberately included some simple illustrations in a 'blackboard' style. At the same time, these illustrations can be used as templates for explaining problems on rounds.

The content reflects the North American experience of the authors. That is, there is heavy emphasis on surgical anatomy and perioperative management. However, all surgeons must be aware of the 'medical' aspects of cardiac and respiratory intensive care, and we have stressed relevant areas of 'non-surgical' ICU care. Similarly, we anticipate that anaesthesiologists or internists (especially in the subspecialties of pulmonary medicine and cardiology) involved in the management of surgical patients desire to have an understanding of relevant surgical issues. The questions, therefore, are designed to be useful across the spectrum of 'surgical' and 'medical' expertise. If we are not to lose sight of the patient underneath all the ICU technology available today, we must strive not to compartmentalize ourselves, but rather broaden our communication and awareness of what all the various specialties have to offer.

Contributors

Mario G. Gasparri, MD
Henry Ford Hospital, Detroit, USA

Benjamin Guslits, MD FRCP
Henry Ford Hospital, Detroit, USA

Andrew Hamilton, MD, FRCS,
    FRCSC(CT)
University of Manitoba, Winnipeg,
Canada

H. Mathilda Horst, MD, FACS, FCCM
Henry Ford Hospital, Detroit, USA

Jay A. Johannigman, MD, FACS
University of Cincinnati, Cincinnati,
USA

Riyad C. Karmy-Jones, MD, FRCSC,
    FRCSC(CT), FCCP
Henry Ford Hospital, Detroit, USA

Arvind Koshal, MD, MBBS, MS,
    FRCSC, FRCSC(CT)
University of Alberta, Edmonton,
Canada

Kurt A. Kralovich, MD
Henry Ford Hospital, Detroit, USA

Catherine LeGalley, MD
Henry Ford Hospital, Detroit, USA

Gordon M. Lees, MD, FRCSC
University of Alberta, Edmonton,
Canada

Joseph W. Lewis Jr., MD, FACS, FCCP
Henry Ford Hospital, Detroit, USA

Cairan J. McNamee, MD, FRCSC
University of Alberta, Edmonton,
Canada

Daniel C. Morris, MD
Henry Ford Hospital, Detroit, USA

John C. Mullen, MD, MSc, FRCSC,
    FRCSC(CT), FCCP, FACS
University of Alberta, Canada

Farouck N. Obeid, MD, FACS
Henry Ford Hospital, Detroit, USA

Iraklis I. Pipinos, MD
Henry Ford Hospital, Detroit, USA

Krishnan Raghavendran, MD
Henry Ford Hospital, Detroit, USA

Fraser D. Rubens, MD, MSc, FRCSC,
    FRCSC(CT)
Ottawa Heart Institute, Ottawa, Canada

Ilan S. Rubinfeld, MD
Henry Ford Hospital, Detroit, USA

Douglas Schuerer, MD
Henry Ford Hospital, Detroit, USA

Vincent A. Simonetti, MD
Wayne State University, Detroit, USA

Victor J. Sorensen, MD, FACS
Henry Ford Hospital, Detroit, USA

Lorie Lee Thomas, PhD
University of Michigan, Ann Arbour,
USA

Eric Vallières, MD, FRCSC
University of Washington, Seattle, USA

James W. Wagner, MD
Henry Ford Hospital, Detroit, USA

Charles R. Webb, MD, FACP, FACC,
    FCCP
Henry Ford Hospital, Detroit, USA

Self-Assessment Color Review of

Cardiothoracic Critical Care

Riyad C. Karmy-Jones
MD, FRCSC, FRCSC(CT), FCCP
Henry Ford Hospital, Detroit, USA

H. Mathilda Horst
MD, FACS, FCCM
Henry Ford Hospital, Detroit, USA

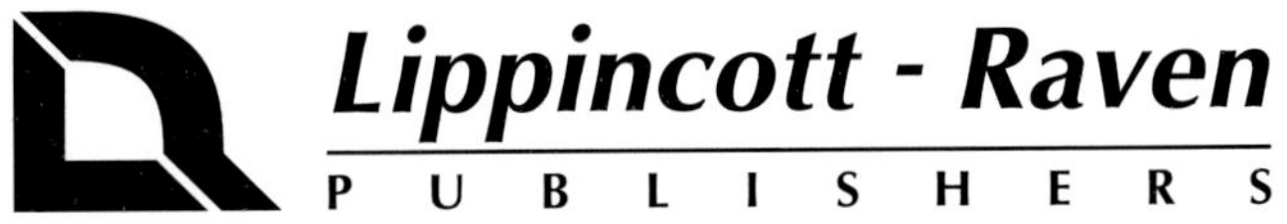

Acknowledgement

We would like to thank Deborah Tredwell for her expert reconstruction of our written work.

Dedications

For Leila and Bill (RKJ)

For Harriette and Walter (HMH)

Published 1998 in North America by:
Lippincott–Raven Publishers,
227 East Washington Square,
Philadelphia, PA 19106–3780
ISBN 0–316–74755–6

Library of Congress Cataloging-in-Publication data applied for.

Typesetting and design: Paul Bennett
Color reproduction: Tenon & Polert Color Scanning Ltd., (HK.)
Printed by: Grafos SA, Barcelona, Spain

Abbreviations

A-kinase adenosine kinase
ABG arterial blood gas
ABI ankle brachial index
ABO blood groups
ABP arterial blood pressure
ACE angiotensin converting enzyme
ACLS advanced cardiac life support
ACT accelerated clotting time
ACTH adrenocorticotrophic hormone
  (corticotrophin)
ADH anti-diuretic hormone
aADO alveolar-arterial O_2 difference
ADP adenosive di-phosphate
AEF aorto-enteric fistula
AI aortic incompetence
AICD automatic internal cardioverter
  defibrillator
Ao aortic
ARDS adult (acute) respiratory distress
  syndrome
ASA acetylsalicylic acid
ASD atrial septal defect
ATLS advanced trauma life support
ATP adenosine 5'-triphosphate
AV atrioventricular
AVA aortic valve area
AVR aortic valve replacement
b.p.m. beats per minute
BO bubble oxygenator
BSA body surface area
CABG coronary artery bypass grafting
cAMP cyclic adenosine 3',5'-phosphate
CASP catheter aspiration
CCS Cardiac Cardiovascular Society
CCU coronary care unit
CDH congenital diaphragmatic hernia
cGMP cyclic guanosine monophosphate
CHF congestive heart failure
CI cardiac index
CMV cytomegalovirus
CNS central nervous system
CO cardiac output
COPD chronic obstructive pulmonary
  disease
CPAP continuous psoitive airway
  pressure

CPB cardiopulmonary bypass
CPK-MB cratine phospotenase-
  myocardial bond
CPR cardiopulmonary resusitation
CSF cerebrospinal fluid
CT computed tomography
CVA cerebral vascular accident
CVP central venous pressure
CXR chest X-ray
DLCO diffusion of carbon monoxide
DDAVP synthetic vasopressin
DIC diffuse intravascular coagulation
DPG diphosphoglyceric acid
DPL diagnostic peritoneal lavage
EBT bay thoracotomy
ECLS extracorrporeal life support
ECMO extracorporeal membrane
  oxygenation
EDP end diastolic pressure
EDV end diastolic volume
EF ejection fraction
EMG electromyogram
EPS exophthalmos-producing substance
ERP effective renal plasma
FEV_1 volume exhaled in first second
FRC functional residual capacity
FVC forced vital capacity
GE gastroesophageal
GI gastrointestinal
GMP guanosine 5'-phosphate
GTP guanosine 5'-triphosphate
HLHS hypoplastic left heart syndrome
IABP intra-aortic balloon pump
ICAM endothelial cell adhesion
  molecule
ICU intensive care unit
IMV intermittent mandatory ventilation
IN isoniazid
INR international normalized ratio
IPA invasive pulmonary aspergillosis
IRV inspiratory reserve volume
IV intravenous
IVC inferior vena cava
LA left atrium
LAD left anterior descending coronary
  artery

LDH lactate dehydrogenase
LIMA left internal mammography
LTB laryngotracheal bronchitis
LTE laryngotracheal-oesophageal
LV left ventricular
MAI mycobacterium avium intracellular
MAC minimal alveolar concentration
MAP mean arterial pressure
MAST military anti-shock trousers
MAT multifocal atrial tachycardia
MI myocardial infarction
MO membrane oxygenator
MOF multiple organ failure
MR mitral regurgitation
MRI magnetic resonance imaging
MVA miltral valve area
MVV maximum voluntary ventilation
NADH/NAD nicotinamide adenine
  dinucleotide
NAPA N-acetyl procainamide
NG nasogastric
NO nitric oxide
NPO nil per ora (nothing by mouth)
NSAID non-steroidal anti-inflammatory
  drug
NYHA New York Heart Association
OR operating room
PA pulmonary artery
PAOC pulmonary artery occlusion
  catheter
PC-IRV inverse ratio pressure control
  ventilation
PCP pneumocystitis with pneumonia
PCWP pulmonary capillary wedge
  pressure
PDA persistent ductus arteriosus
PEEP positive end-expiratory pressure
PFC persistent fetal circulation
PFO patent foramen ovale
PFT pulmonary funtin tests
PMN polymorphonucleocyte
  (neutrophil)
PND paroxysmal nocturnal dyspnoea
PO per ora (by mouth)
PTCA percutaneous tranluminal
  coronary angioplasty

PTFE polytetrafluoroethylene
PTT partial thromboplastin time
PV pulmonary vein
PVC premature ventricular constriction
PVR pulmonary vascular resistence
PR wave
QRS wave
R-on-T waves
RBBB right bundle branch block
RCA right coronary artery
RTA road traffic accident
RV right ventricular
RVH right ventricular hypertrophy
RVOTO right ventricular outflow tract
  obstruction
RR wave
SAM systolic anterior motion
SAT saturation
SBE subacute bacterial endocarditis
SIADH syndrome of inappropriate anti-
  diuretic hormone production
SICU surgical ICU
SVC superior vena cava
SVR systemic vascular resistance
SVT supraventricular tachyarrhythmias
TB tuberculosis
TEG thromboelectrogram
TGA transposition of great arteries
THAM trimethamine
TIF tracheoinnominate fistula
TOF tetralogy of Fallot
tPA tissue plasminogen activator
TPN triphosphopyridine nucleotide
TSH thyroid stimulating hormone
TT thrombin time
VATS video-assisted thorascopic
  surgery
VF ventricular fibrillation
VQ ventricular refusion
VSD ventricular septal defect
VT ventricular tachyarrhythmias
VV veno-venous
WBC white blood cell
WPW Wolf–Parkinson–White

1 This patient presented after suffering extensive burns in a house fire (1). On the second day of hospitalization, he developed severe GI bleeding that required colectomy. In the hours following surgery, it was noted that there was progressive difficulty in ventilating, increasing inotropic requirements and decreasing urine output despite high filling pressures. His abdomen was closed using interrupted stainless steel wires. What should be done next?

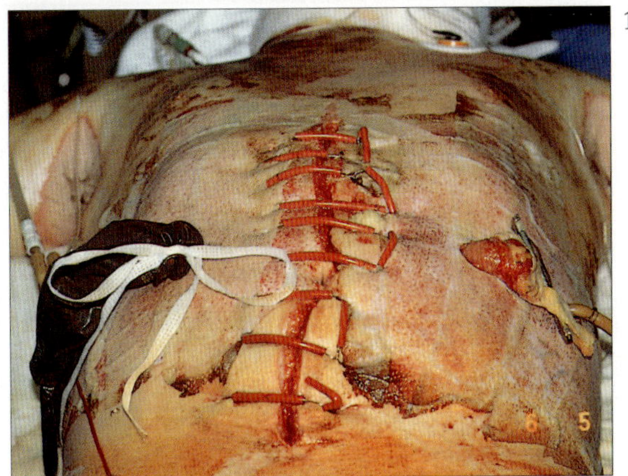

2 In this graph of the oxyhaemoglobin dissociation curve (2), which point represents the P_{50}?
i. A.
ii. B.
iii. C.
iv. D.

3 A 19-year-old is struck by a car while crossing the street. Radiography demonstrated non-displaced right tibia and fibula fractures. Three hours after his arrival, he begins to complain of worsening pain in the leg. He is also noted to have intact pulses with pain to passive motion at the ankle. What is the next step in evaluating/treating this patient?
i. Place ice bags on his leg and elevate to decrease swelling.
ii. Apply a plaster cast to immobilize the extremity.
iii. Obtain an EMG to rule out tibial nerve injury.
iv. Perform compartment pressure measures in all four compartments of the lower leg.

1 Abdominal compartment syndrome results from increased intra-abdominal pressure that leads to obstruction of urine flow and renal arterial supply, decreased preload due to caval occlusion, increased afterload and restrictive pulmonary defects. It can be diagnosed by measuring intra-abdominal pressure, via Foley or NG catheters, although these are variable depending on the position of the patient and method used. Adverse changes may be seen at a pressure >15mmHg (2.0 kPa); a pressure of >30 mmHg (4.0 kPa) is associated with significant effects. If suspected, management includes reopening the abdomen to release pressure. A silo may be needed until swelling decreases. This patient had his midline closed with steel retention sutures, which are associated with the least dehiscence in burn patients. Loosening of the retention decreased the abdominal pressure.

2 B. The oxyhaemoglobin dissociation curve describes the affinity of haemoglobin for oxygen. The oxyhaemoglobin dissociation curve is a sigmoid-shaped curve where under conditions of constant temperature and pH, the haemoglobin saturation can be plotted from the PO_2. Under normal conditions, a PO_2 of 100 mmHg (13.3 kPa) implies 100% saturation. A PO_2 of 60 mmHg (8.0 kPa) implies 85% saturation. The P_{50} describes the position on the curve where haemoglobin is 50% saturated with oxygen. The P_{50} is normally 27 mmHg (3.6 kPa). The position of P_{50} on the oxyhaemoglobin dissociation curve changes with alterations in the temperature, CO_2, Na^+, K^+, H^+ ion concentration, 2,3-DPG and ATP.

3 iv. This patient has early signs of a lower leg compartment syndrome. Immediate measurement of his pressures is necessary to determine the need for fasciotomy. In a patient with more advanced signs, such as weakness of the extensor hallucis longus muscle, decreased sensation over the first web space of the foot, or changes in the pulses at the ankle, a high index of suspicion must be maintained and early fasciotomy is necessary to prevent ischaemic (Volkmann's) contractures. The most common causes of compartment syndrome are divided into those that cause an increase in compartment volume and those that decrease compartment size. Those that increase compartment volume are: post-ischaemic swelling (such as following an arterial occlusion or injury), arterial haemorrhage, soft-tissue crush, fractures with swelling and bleeding, and post-exertional swelling. Those that constrict the compartment include constrictive dressings or casts and burn injury with resultant eschar which limits swelling of the injured muscle. The compartment pressure is measured by using a direct measurement device, such as needle and pressure transducer or the Stryker brand instrument. Normal compartment pressures range from 15–25 mmHg (2.0–3.3 kPa). When the compartment pressure reaches 30–40 mmHg (4.0–5.3 kPa), it is recommended that full fasciotomy of all involved compartments be performed.

4 The CT scan (4) was obtained in a 65-year-old woman with back pain. At admission the blood pressure was 190/110 mmHg (25.3/14.6 kPa). Other physical findings were normal. The most likely cause of her symptom is:
i. Renal calculi.
ii. Aortic dissection.
iii. Aortic aneurysm.
iv. Diaphragmatic hernia.
The management should include:
i. Immediate surgery.
ii. Upper GI series.
iii. Surgery if unable to control blood pressure and/or pain.
iv. IV pyelogram.

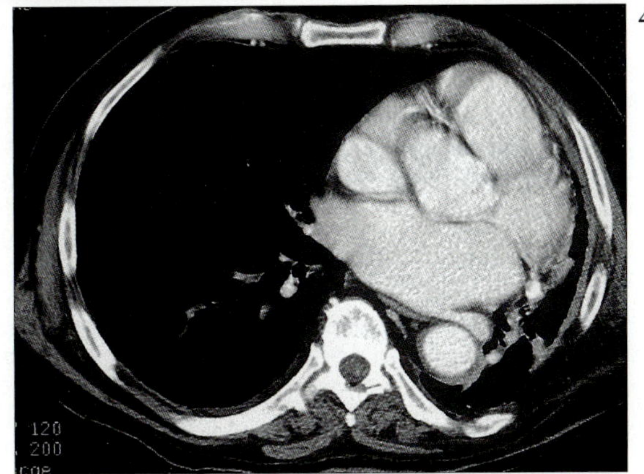

5 An illustration of an action potential of a myocardial cell (5).
i. What do the 'phases' represent?
ii. Which phase correlates with the QRS complex on the ECG?

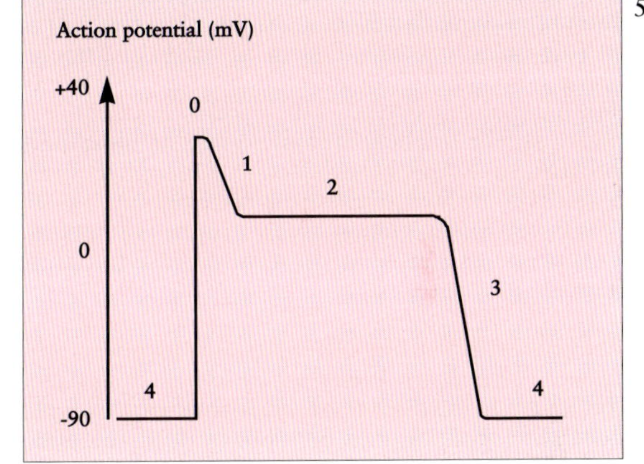

6 Briefly discuss the aetiology of TIF. What diagnostic steps should be taken in a patient with a tracheostomy who is noted to have increasing amounts of blood on suctioning?

7 True or false? Endotracheal drug administration is as effective as IV administration.

4 The CT scan shows a Type B aortic dissection. (There is a faint transverse line in the descending aorta.) Initial treatment is medical and is aimed at reducing the mean arterial pressure and myocardial contractility by using beta blockade and/or unloading agents such as nitroprusside.

The goal of medical therapy is to relieve pain within 4–6 h, control blood pressure and arrest the dissecting process. Failure of medical therapy, that is, inability to control pain or hypertension or evidence of progressive dissection – and signs of impending rupture such as blood in pleura or pericardial effusion – are indications for urgent surgery.

5 Phase 0 represents depolarization, with opening of the fast Na^+ and K^+ channels. This phase correlates with the QRS complex on an ECG. Closure of the Na^+ channels initiates a return towards 0, initiating repolarization (Phase 1). During Phase 2 (correlating with the ST segment of the ECG) Ca^{2+} enters through slow channels. During Phase 3, K^+ efflux returns the membrane potential back to -90 mV, but the normal ionic gradient is not achieved until Phase 4, when the active Na^+–K^+ pump exchanges Na^+ for K^+.

6 TIF occurs when ischaemia results in breakdown of the trachea, usually along the inner curve of the TT, in the area of the innominate artery. Risk factors include low placement (below the fourth ring), prolonged ventilation, and coagulopathy.

A herald bleed occurs in 50% of cases. Work-up consists of examining the tracheal stoma to ensure that bleeding is not from the skin edge, and fibre-optic bronchoscopy to rule out other causes such as tracheitis, pneumonia and suction trauma. If no lesion is found on bronchoscopy that can explain the bleeding, then the possibility of TIF must be considered. This necessitates exploration in the operating room to rule out a deeper tracheal stomal source of bleeding (usually erosion into the thyroid isthmus) and rigid bronchoscopy. Often, TIF still cannot be totally ruled in or out. Surgical control requires median sternotomy.

CT scan and angiography are usually not helpful. CT may suggest loss of the fat or tissue planes between the innominate and trachea,and/or new air along the innominate artery.

7 Endotracheal drug administration is not as effective as IV injection. The effectiveness of endotracheally administered drugs depends on the absorbant surface of the lungs. In cardiac arrest situations with complicating factors such as pulmonary oedema, aspiration and pulmonary flow, the effectiveness of endotracheal drugs is limited. It may be that at least 10 times the currently recommended dose is required.

8 The following cardiac catheterization data were obtained from a 2-year-old infant (numbers are $O_2\%$ saturation) (8). What is the shunt (given a HgB of 10)?

1   78
2   88
3   83
4   88

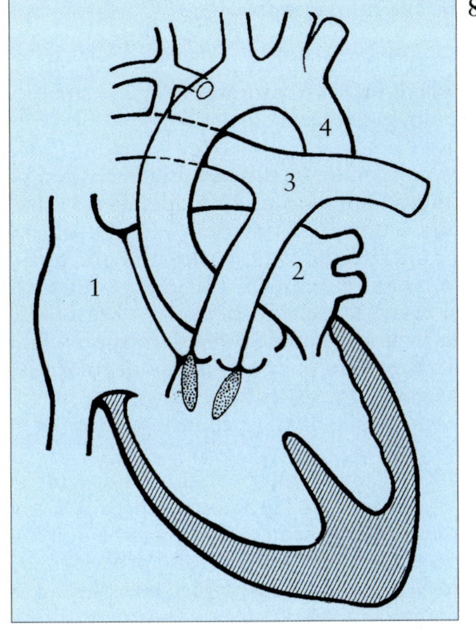

9 What is 'automaticity' and which portion of the heart is characterized by this property?

10 The risk of death with completion pneumonectomy is the highest with which of the following?
i. Benign lung disease.
ii. Lung cancer.
iii. Pulmonary metastases.

11 A 55-year-old man with a nonresectable mid-tracheal tumour developed hypotension and desaturation while undergoing rigid bronchoscopy and attempted dilation. Rapid examination reveals diminished breath sounds bilaterally, and the bronchoscopist feels that the trachea, in the area of the tumour, was perforated. Bilateral chest tubes relieve the pneumothoraces, but the air way collapses whenever the scope is removed. Which of the following would be the most appropriate approach?
i. Emergency tracheal resection.
ii. Laser resection of the tumour.
iii. External stenting of the trachea and mediastinal washout.
iv. Place a stent across the lesion.

8 The ratio of pulmonary (Qp) to systemic flow (Qs), or shunt, can be calculated by:

$$Qp/Qs = (Aosat - SVCsat)/(PVsat - PAsat)$$

where sat = O_2 saturation, SVC = superior vena cava, PV = pulmonary vein and PA = pulmonary artery.

9 Automaticity is noted in specialized conducting cells, in particular those grouped in the SA node and AV node. These cells have a lower membrane permeability to K^+, and a higher resting permeability to Ca^{2+}. This results in a slow spontaneous membrane depolarization which characterises cells with automaticity. When threshold potential is reached, Phase 0 is initiated. In the SA and AV nodes, Phase 0 reflects slower Ca^{2+} entry and is less steep than other myocardial cells. Adrenergic activity hastens spontaneous depolarization while vagal activity decreases it. The SA node has a faster rate of spontaneous depolarization and therefore controls the rate of those automatic cells 'further down the line'. If there should be SA dysfunction, the AV node can 'kick in' at an intrinsic rate of 40–60 b.p.m.

10 i. Completion pneumonectomy for benign disease carries the highest risk, in one series being 28%, as opposed to 9% for lung cancer and 0% for pulmonary metastases. The reason is that most benign lung diseases that require completion pneumonectomy are inflammatory processes, with resultant intense fibrotic hilar changes resulting in increased bleeding, stump problems and infection. All patients undergoing completion pneumonectomy should have the bronchial stump reinforced with a viable tissue pedicle.

11 iv. The most reasonable approach is to stent the lesion, thus maintaining airway patency while closing of the site of perforation. Antibiotics to cover oral flora should be used.

The majority, but not all, of tracheal cancers are unresectable. They may present with the diagnosis of 'asthma', and the use of steroids may complicate surgery. Palliative management includes stenting, dilation, radiation and in critical airway narrowing laser or 'coring out' with a rigid scope. If the airway diameter was less than 6 mm, hyperventilation will be needed once dilation has been accomplished to wash out retained CO_2.

12 What are the risk factors for PA rupture from a PAOC?

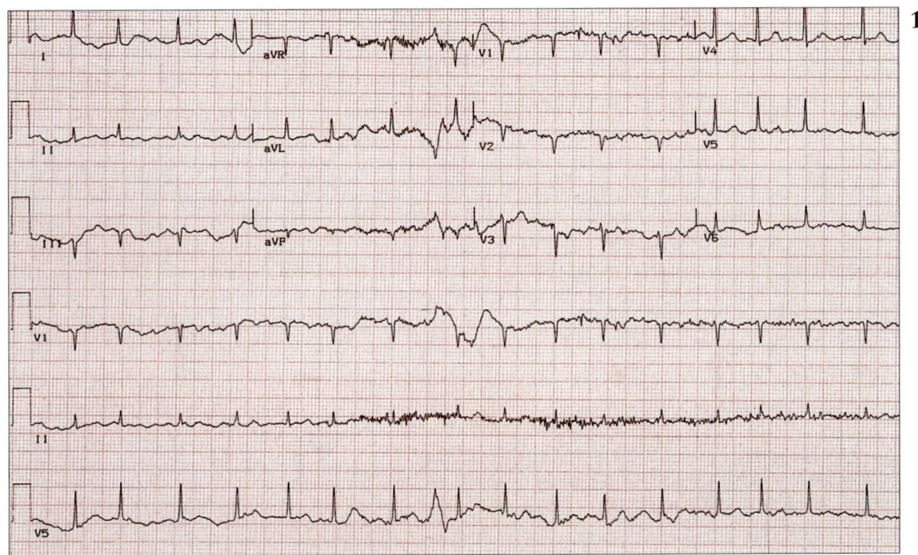

13 A patient is troubled by chronic palpitations and syncopal episodes. His history is significant for peptic ulcer disease. His ECG during one of the episodes is shown (**13**). Discuss the possible surgical management of this patient.

14 List the normal values of the following in an adult:

1. O_2 consumption.
2. $AVDO_2$.
3. CI.
4. SVR.
5. PVR.
6. AVA.
7. MVA.
8. LV EDV.
9. EF.
10. Mean RA pressure.
11. RV systolic pressure.
12. RV EDP.
13. PA mean pressure.
14. PA wedge pressure.
15. LA mean pressure.
16. LV systolic pressure.
17. LV EDP.

15 What effect does neck flexion and extension have on the position of an endotracheal tube?

12 Risk factors include pulmonary hypertension, coagulopathy, advanced age, advancing the catheter too far out into the pulmonary circuit and/or overinflation of the balloon. This has been noted to occur in patients following CPB because of lung deflation and hypothermia which stiffens the catheter and 'pushes' the catheter farther out into the pulmonary vessels than it was when originally placed. It is important to look for the 'overwedge' wave form.

13 Atrial fibrillation is characterized by irregularly irregular rhythm, with no detectable P wave. In chronic atrial fibrillation ventricular response can be controlled with digoxin, beta-blockers, and/or calcium channel blockers. However, anticoagulation is required because of the risk of thromboembolism. In patients whose ventricular rates cannot be controlled, or who suffer significant symptoms, radioablation of the bundle of His followed by pacemaker placement is an option, but also requires anticoagulation. Because atrial fibrillation is believed to be a phenomenon of macro-re-entry circuits, various isolation procedures have been developed, culminating in the 'maze' procedure. This involves resecting and re-anastomosing the atria so as to direct electrical activity from SA node to AV node and to interrupt the macro circuits. It can be performed at the time of other cardiac operations, and long term anticoagulation is not required.

14 1. O_2 consumption = 110–150 ml/min/m^2
2. AVDO$_2$ = 3.5–4.7 vol%
3. CI = 2.5–4.0 l/min/m^2
4. SVR = 8.0–15.0 Wood units (dynes/s/cm^5)
5. PVR = 0.2–1.12 Wood units (dynes/s/cm^5)
6. AVA = 2.6–3.5 cm^2
7. MVA = 4.0–6.0 cm^2
8. LV EDV = <90 ml/m^2
9. EF = 55–70%
10. Mean RA pressure = 1–8 mmHg (0.1–1.1 kPa)
11. RV systolic pressure = 15–28 mmHg (2.0–3.7 kPa)
12. RV EDP = 0–8 mmHg (0–1.1 kPa)
13. PA mean pressure = 10–22 mmHg (1.3–2.9 kPa)
14. PA wedge pressure = 4–12 mmHg (0.5–1.6 kPa)
15. LA mean pressure = 4–12 mmHg (0.5–1.6 kPa)
16. LV systolic pressure = 85–150 mmHg (11.3–20.0 kPa)
17. LV EDP = 4–12 mmHg (0.5–1.6 kPa)

15 With flexion, the endotracheal tube can rise up to 2 cm, as compared with the head in neutral position. With extension it can advance 2 cm.

16 Match the drug with its side effect:

i. Hydralazine.
ii. Esmolol.
iii. Enalaprilat.
iv. Nitroprusside.
v. Adenosine.

a. Angio-oedema.
b. Metabolic acidosis.
c. Asystole.
d. Bronchospasm.
e. Tachycardia.

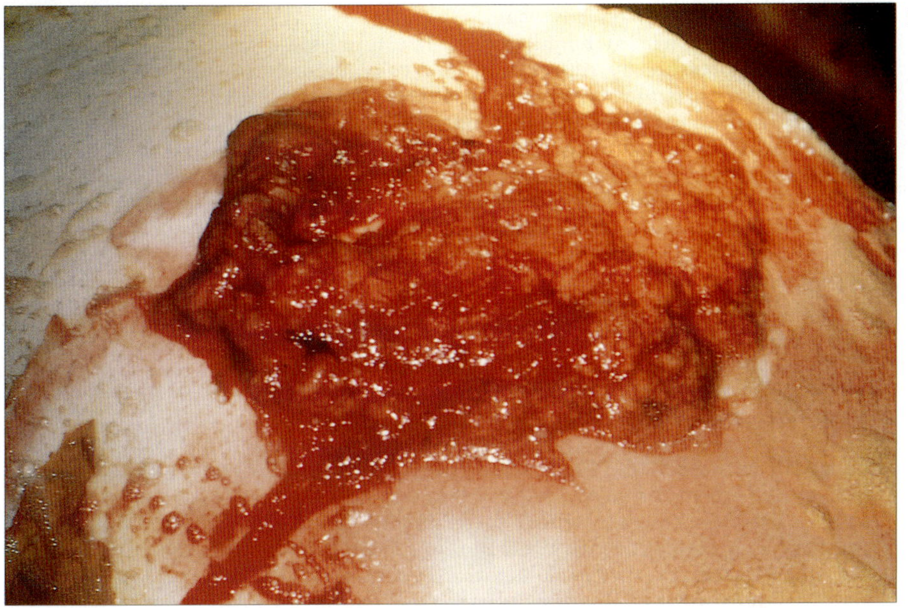

17

17 This 51-year-old man was injured when a parcel device exploded (**17**). Injuries included second and third degree burns of the upper torso, as well as evisceration. Discuss the work-up and management of potential thoracic injuries.

18 True or false? The outcome after cardiac arrest in the paediatric population is better than that in the adult population.

16 i and e; ii and d; iii and a; iv and b; v and c.

Hydralazine is a potent arterial vasodilator. It causes marked decrease of mean ABP and SVR. Hydralazine increases CO and heart rate with the major side effects of tachycardia and headaches. This drug must be used with caution in patients with angina, myocardial infarction and aortic dissection.

Esmolol is a β_1 selective beta-blocker which has a very short duration of action. It is used to control supraventricular tachycardias and has been used to control post-operative hypertension. Severe hypotension is the most common adverse side effect seen, however, in patients with bronchospastic disease, because this is a β_1 selective blocker, it can increase bronchospasm.

Enalaprilat is a potent ACE inhibitor which can be used to control hypertension. It reduces blood pressure by suppressing the renin–angiotensin–aldosterone system. Severe hypotension is the most common adverse side effect seen. Patients receiving this medication can develop angio-oedema.

Nitroprusside is a vasodilator. Nitroprusside is metabolised to thiocyanate. Toxicity symptoms are mental status changes, nausea, abdominal pain, tinnitus, hyper-reflexia and seizures. Cyanide toxicity can also occur and is manifested by metabolic acidosis as well as shortness of breath, headache, vomiting, dizziness, and loss of consciousness. Cyanide toxicity may also be associated with absent reflexes, dilated pupils and a pink colour.

Adenosine is used to diagnose and treat supraventricular dysrhythmias: it can be associated rarely with complete heart block or even asystole.

17 Injuries following explosions can be ascribed to primary, secondary, tertiary and miscellaneous mechanisms. Primary blast injury refer to the effects of the blast wave. Secondary injuries are those caused by flying debris while tertiary refer to injuries sustained if and when the victim is thrown against hard objects. Miscellaneous injuries include thermal and inhalational injuries.

Pulmonary blast injury is similar to pulmonary contusion and ARDS. Alveolar–pulmonary vein fistulation can occur leading to air emboli when positive pressure ventilation is used. Treatment is supportive, and may include hyperbaric oxygenation. These abnormal connections usually 'seal' within 24 h. As the most common injuries among survivors of bomb explosions are thermal and/or orthopaedic, if such a pulmonary insult is suspected, general anaesthesia, positive pressure ventilation and operations should be delayed during this period if possible.

Auditory findings should indicate a risk for primary blast injury.

Other possible pulmonary injuries include inhalational burns and/or frank contusion. These are managed supportively with avoidance of excessive fluid (if possible), physiotherapy and ventilatory support as needed. The possibility of blunt cardiac injury ('contusion') should also be considered.

18 False. Cardiac arrest in paediatric patients is more commonly bradycardic or asystolic arrest than VF. It is often related to respiratory problems. The adult arrest victim, because of the acute onset of VF which rapidly responds to defibrillation, tends to have an improved outcome.

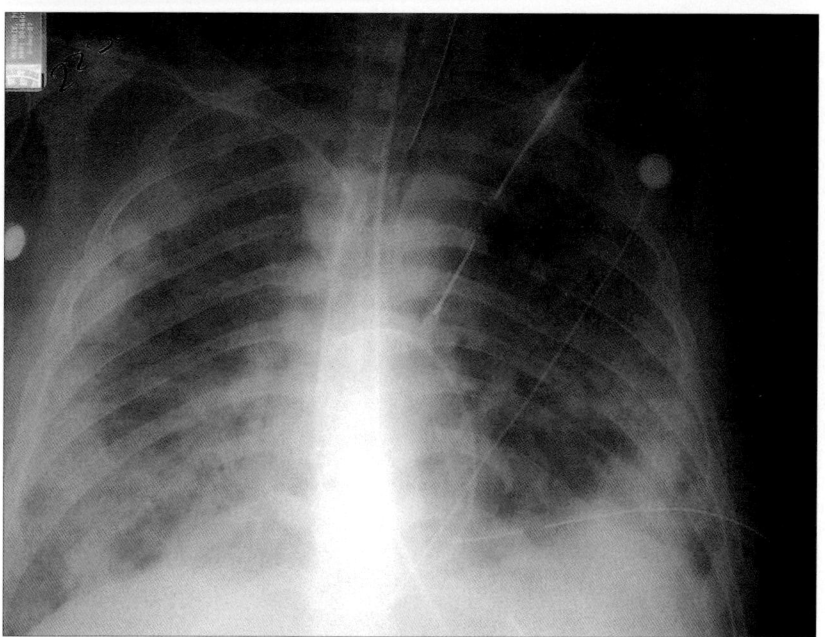

19 A 72-year-old man presented to the emergency department with respiratory failure secondary to pneumonia (**19**). He needed intubation with mechanical ventilation and inotropic support was required to maintain haemodynamic stability. His clinical course was complicated by the development of a parapneumonic effusion. A thoracentesis was performed. Indications for chest tube drainage include:
i. Pleural fluid glucose of 80 mg/dl (8 mg/ml).
ii. Pleural fluid pH of 7.21 ($[H^+] = 60$).
iii. Pleural fluid LDH of 100 IU/l.
iv. Pleural fluid Gram stain showing Gram-positive cocci in chains.

20 After termination of CPB following a quadruple aortocoronary bypass operation and protamine administration, the patient shows widening of the QRS complex, blood pressure 80/50 mmHg (10.6/6.7 kPa). PA pressures 54/28 mmHg (7.2/3.7 kPa) (mean 34 mmHg (4.5 kPa)) and a pulse rate of 60 b.p.m.
    Management should include one or more of the following:
i. Administration of adrenaline.
ii. Reheparinization and resumption of CPB.
iii. Give agents to reduce PVR.
iv. Give a second dose of protamine.

21 What is the difference between 'automaticity' and 're-entry'?

19 ii and iv. Parapneumonic effusions occur in up to 50% of patients requiring hospitalization for community-acquired pneumonia. The utility of pleural fluid pH, lactate dehydrogenase and glucose in identifying complicated parapneumonic effusions that require drainage remains controversial. A recent meta-analysis found that pleural fluid pH had the highest diagnostic accuracy for all patients with parapneumonic effusions compared to glucose and LDH. Pleural fluid pH retained its diagnostic accuracy even after excluding patients with purulent effusions. The threshold of pleural fluid pH varied between 7.21 and 7.29 depending on cost-prevalence considerations. A pH of 7.29 ($[H^+] = 51$) was considered the decision threshold for determining the need for chest tube drainage in patients with a high clinical suspicion of pleural infection. For low-risk patients, the threshold was a pH of 7.21 ($[H^+] = 60$).

20 i, ii and iii. Protamine reaction must be considered in unexplained post-bypass hypotension especially in a patient who has received protamine or has taken protamine containing insulin or is allergic to shellfish or who has undergone vasectomy. Rapid administration of protamine produces hypotension by generalised vasodilatation. Protamine can cause acute pulmonary vasoconstricton with right heart failure and bronchospasm mediated by thromboxane release induced by heparin protamine complexes.

The treatment of protamine reaction includes restoring circulation by use of adrenaline and if necessary reheparinizing to CPB. PVR can be lowered by agents such as isoproterenol, nitroglycerine, or prostaglandin E. The actual incidence of true protamine reaction is about 1%. Persistent bradycardia would require temporary pacing.

21 Tachyarrhythmias may be related to increased 'automaticity' or 're-entrant'. Automaticity is a result of a focal area(s) setting of independent signals. Often the underlying aetiology is metabolic, including hypokalaemia, hypocalcaemia, hypoxia and increased adrenaline. Re-entrant tachyarrhythmias are created when two possible pathways exist to conduct impulses, one capable of conducting only retrograde. If an impulse is carried through one limb, and the refractory period of the pathways are such that repolarization occurs in time to allow retrograde conduction through the second limb, a cycle of stimuli can be set up, resulting in a re-entry tachyarrhythmia.

22 Discuss the management of haemoptysis associated with PAOC trauma in cardiac patients in the following settings:
i. Intra-operatively, after induction and placement of the catheter, but prior to incision.
ii. Intra-operatively, before institution of bypass.
iii. Postoperatively.

23 A patient, whose chest radiograph is shown (**23**), had a tracheostomy placed two months previously because of ventilator dependence following a significant stoke. During suctioning several hundred ml of bright blood was noted in the tube. Discuss the management of the patient.

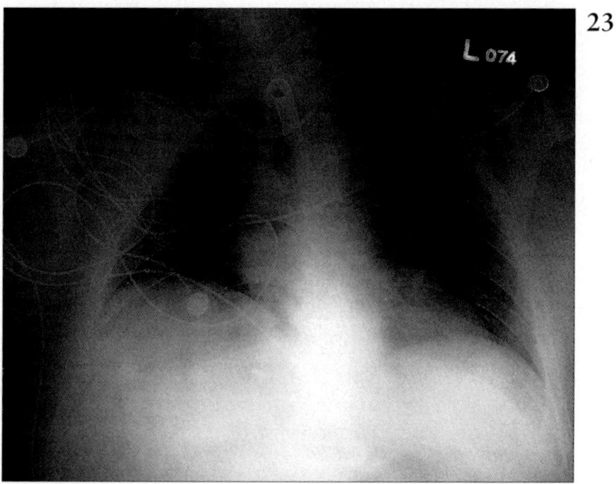

23

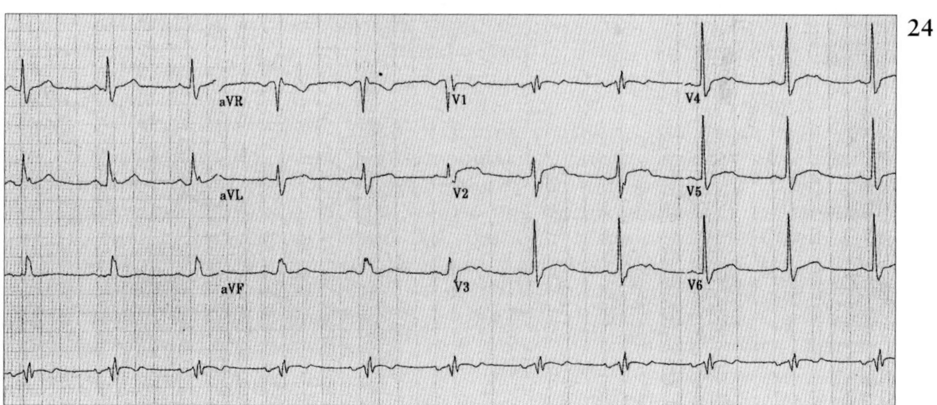

24

24 What is the conduction abnormality in this ECG (**24**)?

22 i. In the post-induction, but preoperative setting, initial management is to prevent 'drowning' of the unaffected lung. The majority of PAOC induced PA ruptures affect the right middle or lower lobes. Quick bronchoscopy followed by placement of an endobronchial blocker will isolate the bleeding site. If the cardiac operation can be postponed, the patient should be monitored in an ICU for 24 h. At the end of that time the blocker is dropped under bronchoscopic examination but the deflated blocker is kept in place and the patient on the ventilator for a further 24 h. If no bleeding has occurred at the end of that time, the patient can be extubated. Serial CXRs should be obtained during this period to make sure that there is no haemothorax that would necessitate thoracotomy. Antibiotics should be given. If haemoptysis recurs during this monitoring period, options include embolization (successful in 70% but with a 30% recurrence rate) or lobectomy. Lobectomy can be performed in the same setting as the cardiac procedure.
ii. If the cardiac operation cannot be delayed, or if haemoptysis occurs while on or about to initiate CPB, the cardiac procedure should be completed. With CPB the lungs are collapsed, which often tamponades the bleeding. Before coming off pump, bronchoscopy (rigid and/or flexible) can be performed with pulmonary isolation. Further, the patient now has a 'better' heart to withstand the stress of having the pulmonary injury dealt with.
iii. Should massive haemoptysis occur postoperatively in the ICU, initial manoeuvres are to place the affected side down, and withdraw the PAOC 1–2 cm and try reinflation in an attempt to occlude the vessel proximally. The remainder of the management is that of acute haemoptysis. Some centres allow only one measurement of the pulmonary occlusion pressure, and then rely on PA pressure alone.

23 When a patient presents with catastrophic bleeding and TIF is suspected, an initial controlling manoeuvre that can be attempted is to hyperinflate the balloon, and pull back and upwards on the tracheostomy tube to occlude the fistula. If this fails, the tube should be removed, a finger inserted into the tracheal lumen and pushed upwards in the region of the innominate, while the patient is reintubated orally with a number 6 endotracheal tube.

Digital control is maintained while sternotomy is performed. Adjunctive measures at this time include type and cross, antibiotics and correcting all coagulation abnormalities. With proximal control of the innominate gained within the pericardium, the fistula can be identified. This may require a probe placed into the trachea. The innominate artery should be ligated and divided, and the tracheal defect repaired and covered with viable tissue (e.g. strap muscle). The innominate should not be reconstructed at that time as the field must be considered contaminated. The majority of patients who survive this catastrophic event curiously do not have any major neurological sequelae from innominate ligation. Consideration can be given to extra-anatomic bypass if needed.

In this case, the patient is moribund with little if any hope of any meaningful recovery in the best of circumstances. A serious consideration should be given by the team and the patient's family to doing nothing.

24 Complete right bundle branch block. Note the RSR complex in lead V1, and large S waves in the lateral leads (V1 and V6). The rhythm is normal sinus with 1:1 correlation of P waves to QRS complexes and a constant PR interval of 190 ms.

25 This patient was admitted after suffering blunt trauma and subsequently developed pneumonia. It is found that when she lies with her left side down, saturations decrease to the mid-80s. They improve when she lies with her right side down. Explain these phenomena.

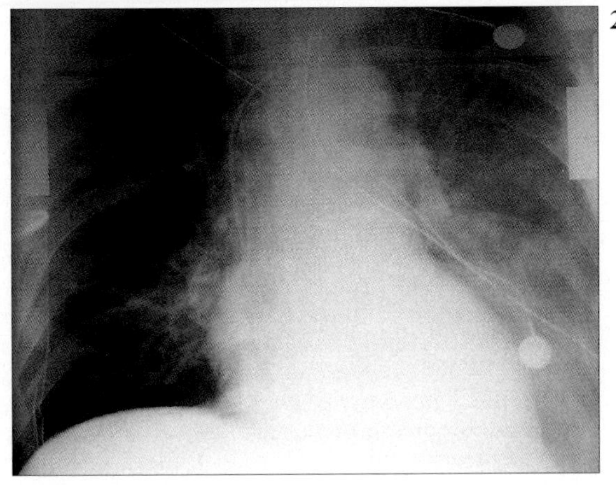

26 A 35-year-old airline pilot presents with WPW syndrome. The best treatment option is:
i. Catheter ablation.
ii. Surgical intervention.
iii. Beta-blockers.
iv. AICD insertion.

27 The tracheobronchial injury from blunt trauma (27) is likely to be:
i. Most commonly transverse and in the cervical trachea?
ii. Most commonly longitudinal and in the left main bronchus?
iii. Most commonly transverse and in the right bronchus?
iv. Most commonly transverse and in the thoracic trachea?

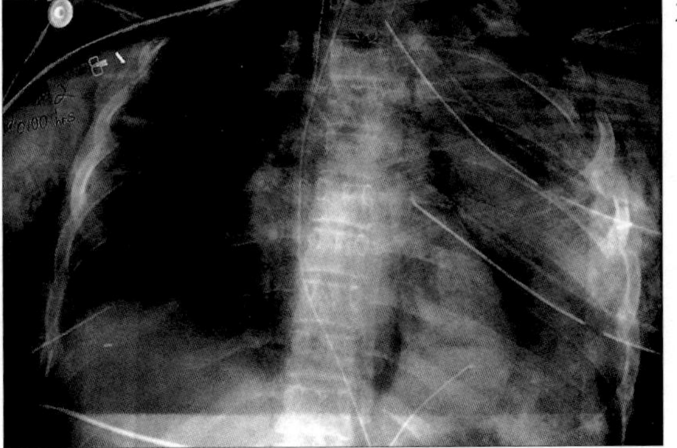

25 When the patient lies on her right, there is preferential flow of blood to the 'uninjured' lung, with better VQ matching. A similar situation can be seen with other causes of unilateral parenchymal disease, such as aspiration. Some patients with diffuse parenchymal disease benefit from being placed on a rotating bed that allows shifting of position at different intervals.

26 i. WPW occurs in 0.25% of patients, three-quarters of whom are asymptomatic. The remainder develop symptoms ranging from palpitations to sudden death. Some congenital heart conditions, notably Ebstein's anomaly, have an increased incidence of WPW (13% in Ebstein's). Sudden death is more common if the refractory period of the accessory pathway is less than 250 ms. These patients are at particular risk from atrial fibrillation because of the possibility of rapid impulse transfer to the ventricle, which degenerates into ventricular fibrillation.

Patients who have experienced sudden death, who have symptoms, or who otherwise are at high risk (athletes, airline pilots, positive family history of sudden death, Ebstein's disease) should undergo evaluation by EPS. Abrupt loss of the accessory pathway with increased heart rates suggest a prolong ERP of the pathway and low risk of ventricular fibrillation. High-risk patients who are asymptomatic but who should be considered for further therapy include the following:

- RR <250 ms during atrial fibrillation.
- ERP of accessory path <250 ms.
- Multiple pathways.
- Need to have cardiac surgery for another reason.

Other patients can be managed by beta-blockers and/or type Ia antidysrhythmics. Catheter ablation is usually successful. Surgical intervention is considered in those patients who have life-threatening symptoms, who have failed radiocatheter ablation or who require cardiac surgery for another reason. Intra-operative mapping is required. The pathways are located in the following sites: left ventricular free wall (60%), posterior septal (20%), right ventricular free wall (10%), anterior septal area (10%). All but the latter can be approached via the epicardial route. The primary advantage is the lack of need to open and therefore arrest the heart as is the case with the endocardial route. The epicardial route may be associated with a higher failure rate however, due to deeper or multiple tracts. The overall success rate is 95%.

27 iii. Bronchogenic tears due to blunt trauma are most commonly transverse and occur in the right main bronchus. Review has shown that these tears are usually transverse 74% of the time versus longitudinal 17%. Of the transverse tears, 4% are in the cervical trachea, 12% are in the thoracic trachea, 25% in the right main bronchus and 17% in the left main bronchus; 16% are in a lobar bronchus.

28 Three patients are being ventilated at tidal volumes of 800 ml, PEEP 5 cm H_2O (28). What do their expiratory pressures suggest?

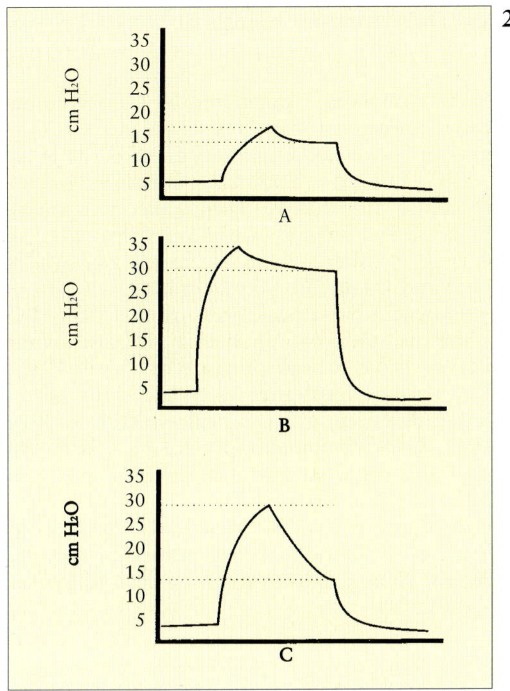

29 What are the 'normal' values for vital signs in paediatric patients in terms of pulse, systolic blood pressure and respiratory rate for:
i. Infants.
ii. Children.
iii. Adolescents?

30 A 45-year-old woman with a life-long history of asthma presents in severe respiratory distress requiring intubation. Physical examination reveals minimal air movement bilaterally with only an occasional wheeze. Arterial blood gas is 65 mmHg (8.7 kPa). The initial ventilator settings are tidal volume 700 ml, 100% oxygen and respiratory rate of 20. Ten minutes after intubation the patient loses her pulse and blood pressure and rhythm strip shows sinus tachycardia with PVCs. Chest radiography shows properly placed endotracheal tube in good position with clear lung fields and no pneumothorax. What action will bring back her pulse and blood pressure?

28 There are three sources of 'resistance': airway resistance (Raw), lung and parenchymal resistance (Rl) and chest wall resistance (Rcw). Static resistance (Rs) is a measure of chest wall and lung resistance while there is no airflow [$Rs = Rc + Rcw$]. Static compliance, calculated by Cs = volume delivered/[plateau pressure - PEEP], is the reciprocal of static resistance ($Cs = 1/Rs$). Dynamic compliance (Cd), which is a measure of overall compliance and is the inverse of total resistance ($Rt = Raw + Rcw + Rl$). Thus $Cd = 1/Rt$ and is measured as: volume delivered/[peak pressure - PEEP]. Dynamic (or effective) compliance is named above because it is a measurement of pressure and volume continuousy through a single breath. Thus differences in Cs and Cd reflect differences in the major airways. Normal values of Cs are 60–100 ml/cm H_2O and Cd are 50–80 ml/cm H_2O.

Patient A has a peak pressure of 15 cm H_2O and a plateau pressure of 13 cm H_2O. Thus the static compliance is 100 and dynamic compliance 80 which are normal. Patient B has a peak pressure of 35 cm H_2O and a plateau pressure of 30 cm H_2O. The static compliance (32) and dynamic compliance (26.6) are both markedly reduced. Patient C has a peak pressure of 30 cm H_2O and plateau pressure of 15 cm H_2O. The dynamic compliance (32) is much more reduced than static compliance (66) and could suggest a mechanical problem such as plugging of the endotracheal tube.

In paediatric units particularly, because of the small volumes delivered, volume lost by ventilator tube expansion can significantly reduce actual delivered volume. Actual volume delivered can be derived by the following formula: True TV = TV – (3 × PIP).

29

	Infants	Children	Adolescents
Heart rate (b.p.m.)	140–160	120–140	90–120
Systolic blood pressure (mmHg (kPa))	80 (10.7)	90 (12.0)	100 (13.3)
Respiratory rate (breaths/min)	35–45	25–35	15–25

30 Turn off the ventilator and readjust the settings to avoid air stacking or 'auto-peep'. Air trapping develops in asthmatic patients who are mechanically ventilated. This patient has severe bronchospasm and small airway obstruction. Time available for expiration should be maximized by reducing respiratory frequency and tidal volume. In severe asthma, the expiration is prolonged and cannot be completed before the next inspiration starts, therefore breaths are 'stacked' and auto-peep develops. In other words, with each subsequent breath, there is a positive end-expiratory alveolar pressure so that PEEP rises. The lung volume due to PEEP increases which increases PVR and RV afterload, decreases in RV afterload causes LV afterload which reduces CO and ABP. Ventilator settings in this patient should be reduced to respiratory rate of 8–10 breaths/min and a tidal volume of 500 ml. Although her $PaCO_2$ will remain elevated, her haemodynamics will stabilize. Bicarbonate can be used to treat cardiac arrhythmias that may develop from her acidosis. Ultimately, her elevated $PaCO_2$ will resolve when her bronchospasm resolves with β_2-agonist bronchodilators and IV corticosteroids. Some centres use aminophylline as a first-use therapy for 'status asthmaticus'. Inhalational ether may also help.

31 A 45-year-old man develops ARDS following a RTA wherein he sustained a closed head injury and multiple long bone fractures (**31**). Pharmacological agents that could be used to treat this patient and have been proven to reduce mortality associated with ARDS include:
i. Exogenous surfactant.
ii. NO.
iii. Prostaglandin E₁.
iv. Corticosteroids.
v. None of the above.

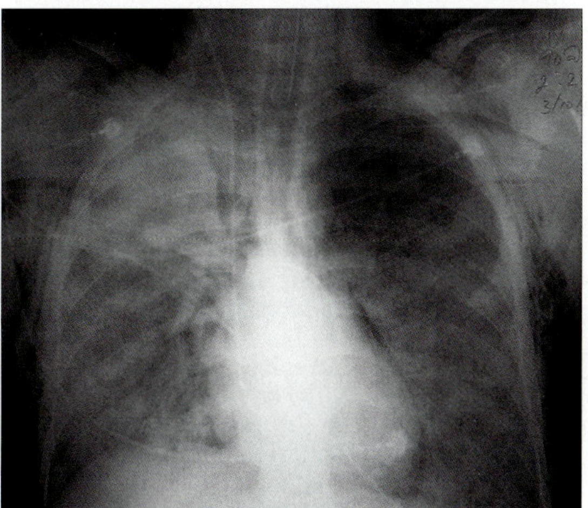

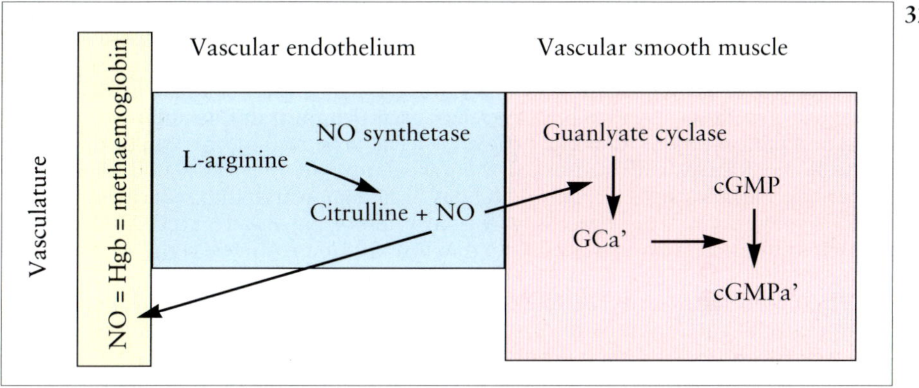

32 The pharmacological pathway of NO in the pulmonary vasculature (**32**).
i. Describe the anticipated pulmonary effects of inhalational NO.
ii. What concentrations are thought to be effective in the treatment of ARDS?
iii. What are the primary toxicity concerns with the administration of NO?

33 Symptomatic bronchogenic cysts in adults are best treated by:
i Observation and antibiotics.
ii. Observation until an air fluid level develops and then sclerosis.
iii. Percutaneous drainage if they are intrapulmonary.
iv. Drainage by mediastinoscopy.
v. Thoracotomy and resection.

31 v. Patients with ARDS have normal amounts of surfactant but it is dysfunctional. Synthetic surfactant has not been reported to have clinical efficacy in ARDS. Inhaled NO is a selective pulmonary vasodilator. NO is an effective agent to reduce the pulmonary hypertension associated with ARDS. However, studies showing the effect of NO on ARDS associated mortality are preliminary. Prostaglandin E_1 blocks platelet aggregation, modulates inflammation and causes vasodilatation. It is effective in alleviating pulmonary hypertension but its use has produced no survival advantage in ARDS. Corticosteroids administered early in the course of ARDS have not reduced mortality and while there is growing popularity to administer corticosteroids to patients in the fibroproliferative phase of the disease, its effect on mortality awaits prospective, blinded, randomized clinical trials.

32 i. NO has been the subject of intense interest in the last five years. Its original description was linked to research investigating the mediation of vascular tone and the description of the substance of the agent called Endothelial Relaxing Factor (EDRF). In 1987, EDRF was identified as NO and demonstrated to be the pathway for agents such as nitroprusside. NO is produced in the vascular endothelium from the cleavage of the N-terminal end of arginine by the enzyme NO synthetase. NO subsequently migrates to adjacent vascular smooth muscle where it effects an increase in cGMP levels via stimulation of guanylate cyclase. Elevation of cGMP levels in vascular smooth muscle produces vasodilatation. The effects of NO are locally limited due to the affinity of NO for haemoglobin with resultant conversion to methaemoglobin.

ii. NO is felt to have at least two important actions in the treatment of ARDS. At extremely low doses (5–50 p.p.b.) NO has been demonstrated to improve oxygenation and reduce venous admixture (Qva/Qt). The presumed mechanism of this effect is by direct, local vasodilatation of the vasculature serving ventilated alveoli. At higher concentrations (1–30 p.p.m.) NO has been demonstrated to reduce pulmonary artery hypertension. This effect is particularly important in advanced ARDS where significant pulmonary artery hypertension often produces right ventricular dysfunction.

iii. The potential toxicity of NO remains to be demonstrated. NIOSH permits exposure to NO at 25 p.p.m. for up to 8 h per day. Therapeutic levels of inhalational NO are thought to be in the range of 1–40 p.p.m. High levels of NO (5,000–20,000 p.p.m.) are associated with hypoxaemia and death. The primary toxicity concern with NO relates to the generation of methaemoglobin and NO_2. The generation of NO_2 may be controlled by limiting circuit time and through the use of lime soda scrubbers. The use of these precautions has limited the measurable NO_2 levels to less than 1 p.p.m.

33 v. The treatment of asymptomatic bronchogenic cysts is still debatable but symptomatic cysts should be treated in a definitive manner. In addition, intrapulmonary cysts tend to have a high incidence of infection and probably should be resected. Aspiration is associated with some recurrence which causes greater difficulty at further surgery and therefore definitive resection is likely better for symptomatic cysts. Sclerosis of cysts with air fluid levels should never be done as these cysts have a connection to the airway.

34 Identify the following channels of the cardiac plasma membrane (34).

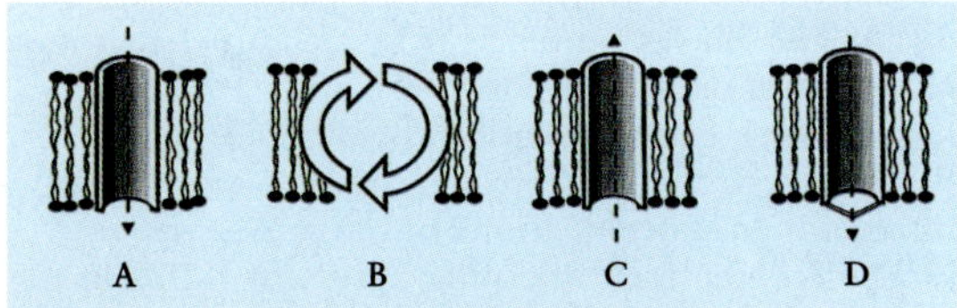

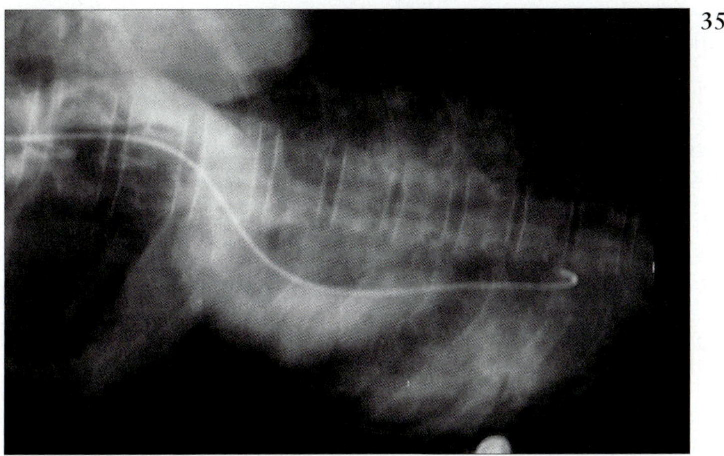

35 A 76-year-old man, with a history of hypertension, presents with back pain, normal ECG, and absent femoral pulses. This aortogram is obtained (35). The patient has significant abdominal tenderness, is acidotic and oliguric, and has a serum lactate that is elevated. Appropriate interventions might include:
i. Palliative care only.
ii. Emergency thoraco-abdominal aortic bypass.
iii. Operative 'fenestration'.
iv. Mini-laparotomy.
v. All of the above.

36 Briefly list the pulmonary manifestation of AIDS.

37 The best overall operative management of benign oesophageal perforations is:
i. Thoracotomy and drainage.
ii. Thoracotomy and resection.
iii. Exclusion and diversion.
iv. Thoracotomy and repair.
v. Conservative management.

34 A The Na$^+$ channel is a fast channel that is controlled by a voltage-dependent gate that is opened by depolarization to allow Na$^+$ entry. It is blocked by lidocaine (lignocaine), quinidine and procainamide.
B The Ca^{2+}/Na$^+$ exchange channel expels either Ca^{2+} or Na$^+$ depending upon intracellular concentrations of the ions.
C The K$^+$ channel, allowing egress of K$^+$ from the cell, is opened by depolarization and closed by repolarization.
D The Ca^{2+} channel is controlled by two gate mechanisms. The outer gate is passive and voltage dependent. The inner gate opens to various degrees depending upon phosphorylation and is therefore mediated by cAMP. This slow channel is the target of the calcium channel blockers.

35 v. This patient with an aortic dissection has evidence of renal and mesenteric ischemia. While aggressive surgical approaches have been tried from time to time, this is usually a nonresuscitatable stage. One option is to do nothing, but if there is some question, mini-laparotomy can confirm ischaemic bowel changes, as well as giving some suggestion as to whether these changes may be reversible with reperfusion. If surgery is entertained, formal thoraco-abdominal grafting may be needed. Occasionally, with a chronic dissection, simply connecting the false and true lumen by creating a 'fenestration' between them may be sufficient.

36 1. Opportunistic pneumonia including PCP, strongyloides, toxoplasmosis. PCP is the initial presentation in 50% of patients and 80% of AIDS patients have at least one episode. In patients who have been treated by aerosolized pentamidine, pneumothoraces are a risk due to necrosis of the lung concomitant with death of the organisms. In patients who have been treated with pentamidine, PCP presents basally whereas in a patient who has not been treated with pentamidine, the PCP presents more often in the upper lobes.
2. Viral pneumonia (commonly CMV).
3. Pyogenic pneumonia.
4. Mycobacterial pneumonia including 'atypical' strains such as MAI and TB.
5. Fungal disease.
6. Pneumothorax related to PCP as mentioned above.
7. Non-infectious complications including Kaposi's sarcoma, lymphoma (diffuse T-cell), lymphocytic pneumonia.
8. Extra-parenchymal manifestations including lymphadenopathy.

37 iv. The best overall approach for benign oesophageal perforation without gross contamination or devitalization of tissue is to repair the oesophagus. The treatment of oesophageal perforation shows the mortality rate of 15% with primary repair, 34% with drainage alone, 29% with resection, 39% with exclusion and diversion and 22% with non-operative management.

38 A 32-year-old man is mechanically ventilated in the ICU following a gunshot wound to the abdomen. His chest radiograph is shown (38). His PaO_2/FiO_2 = 150 mmHg (20.0 kPa) on 17 cm H_2O PEEP and 60% oxygen. His PA wedge pressure is 18 mmHg (2.4 kPa). The patient has:
i. CHF.
ii. Acute lung injury syndrome.
iii. Pulmonary embolism.
iv. ARDS.

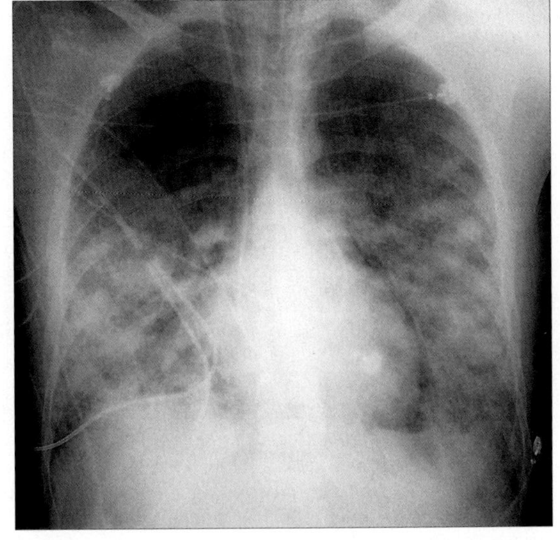

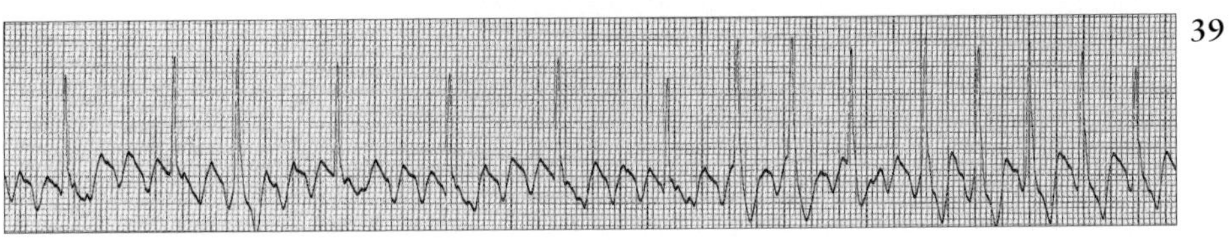

39 A postoperative mitral valve repair ECG.
i. What is the rhythm?
ii. What is the approximate atrial rate?
iii. What is the approximate ventricular rate and does it vary?

40 What abnormalities may be associated with the DiGeorge syndrome?

41 Describe the presentation of acute epiglottitis in a 4-year-old boy and a 23-year-old man.

38 iv. The American–European consensus conference on ARDS defined acute lung injury as having an acute onset, a deterioration in oxygenation with a PaO_2/FiO_2 <300 mmHg (40 kPa) (where PaO_2 is in mmHg (kPa)) regardless of PEEP level, bilateral infiltrates on frontal chest radiograph, and a PA wedge pressure <18 mmHg (2.4 kPa). ARDS was also defined as a disease with acute onset, bilateral infiltrates on frontal chest radiograph, and a PA wedge pressure <18 mmHg (2.4 kPa). However, for ARDS, the PaO_2/FiO_2 must be <200 mmHg (27 kPa) regardless of PEEP level.

39 i. Atrial flutter with variable ventricular rates.
ii. The atrial rate is 300 b.p.m. which is typical for flutter.
iii. Initially there is a physiologic (protective) 4:1 block in the AV node with a resultant ventricular rate of about 85 b.p.m., but this is variable. At the end of the tracing the block is 2:1 and the resultant ventricular rate is 150 b.p.m.

40 DiGeorge syndrome is associated with congenital heart disease including coarctation, interrupted aorta, right sided arch, aortic stenosis, pulmonary atresia and/or TOF. Patients may also present with tetany secondary to hypoparathyroidism. The associated thymic hypoplasia results in decreased cell-mediated immunity and places the patient at risk for fungal, viral and protozoal infections, in particular pneumocystitis pneumonia. Some patients also have a broader immunoglobulin deficiency.

41 The 4-year-old boy will present in the typical classical form of rapid onset of respiratory distress with stridor, fever (39–40°C) and a toxic appearance. The child sits up with his head extended with drooling and speaks with a muffled voice. The child will have been ill less than 24 h and coughing is rare. Children less than 24 months present atypically. Coughing is present in 50% and most are not toxic appearing. Few children in this group prefer the sitting position and most have a normal voice. Drooling is present in only 50% of cases and 25% are afebrile. Adults usually present 1–2 days after the onset of illness, with one-third presenting at least 4 days after onset of symptoms. The majority of adults present with dysphagia and sore throat. Fever is absent in up to one-third of patients and a voice change is present in over half. The diagnosis is often delayed in adults because most complain of sore throat and dysphagia and do not have signs of airway obstruction. Epiglottitis should be suspect in those adult patients who complain of sore throat but have a normal oropharyngeal examination, muffled voice or drooling. Finally, adults differ from children in that the inflammation is not confined to the epiglottis (as in children) but can also affect other structures, such as the pharynx, uvula, base of the tongue, aryepiglottic folds and false vocal cords.

42 A 63-year-old patient presents to the SICU with a temperature of 39°C, lactic acidosis and a rigid abdomen. The chest radiograph shows free air under the diaphragm. The diagram represents the oxyhaemoglobin dissociation curve (**42**). Which curve represents this patient?

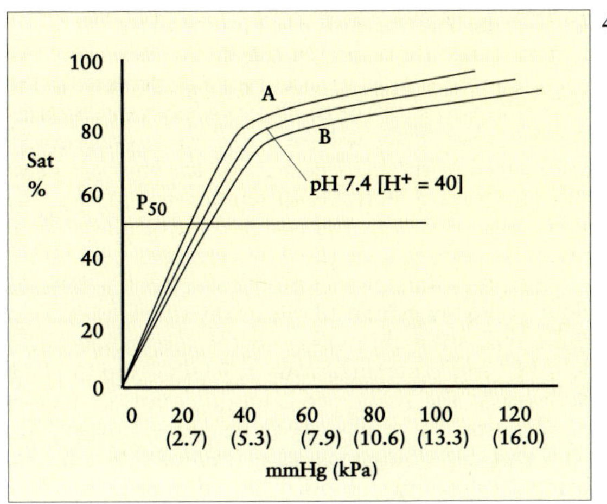

43 A 70-year-old woman with calcific mitral valve stenosis undergoing mitral valve replacement develops a sudden gush of blood from the posterior aspect of the heart following discontinuation of CPB. It appears that the patient has an AV rupture. Management should include:
i. Initiation of protamine administration and fresh frozen plasma.
ii. Elevating the heart and repairing the posterior rupture by mattress sutures.
iii. Institution of CPB, removal of the prosthesis and intraventricular repair.
iv. Institution of CPB and using fibrin glue to seal the site of rupture.

44 Discuss the management options when confronted with a stable 28-year-old woman, who is 24 weeks pregnant, and has a documented descending thoracic aortic tear following blunt trauma.

42 Curve B represents the patient. The P_{50} is affected by multiple factors. These factors cause the value of the P_{50} to increase or decrease, thereby shifting the oxy-haemoglobin dissociation curve. An increase in the P_{50} to a value of over 27 mmHg (3.6 kPa) will shift the oxyhaemoglobin dissociation curve to the right. On this right-shifted curve, there will be a decrease in haemoglobin affinity for O_2. Factors which are related to the increased P_{50} or the shift of the oxyhaemoglobin dissociation curve to the right are increases in temperature, CO_2, Na^+, K^+, H^+ ion concentration, 2,3-DPG and ATP. This right-shifted curve allows increased oxygen release to the tissue level. A decrease in the P_{50} to values less than 27 mmHg (3.6 kPa) shifts the oxyhaemoglobin dissociation curve to the left. This left-shifted curve implies that there is less oxygen available at the tissue level. Factors which decrease the P_{50} or shift the oxyhaemoglobin curve to the left include decreases in temperature, CO_2, Na^+, K^+, H^+ ion concentration, 2,3-DPG and ATP. In efforts to improve oxygen on delivery at the tissue level, modification of factors that affect the oxyhaemoglobin dissociation curve have been attempted mainly through regulation of temperature, CO_2 and $[H^+]$. Surgeons have attempted to adjust this curve in the trauma patient by using fresh whole blood. This eliminates the factor of temperature and 2,3-DPG which are affected by using banked blood.

43 iii. Ventricular rupture occurs in approximately 1% of patients having mitral valve replacement. The outcome of the rupture, once it happens, will probably be fatal. Predisposing factors are small atrium, elderly patients with advanced heart disease and patients with calcific mitral annulus or degenerative disease of the mitral valve. Elevating the heart once the valve is in can predispose to intra-operative injury.

Several methods of repair are available. Repair should preferably be done using a patch. When the opening is in the AV groove or nearby, an intraventricular repair technique should be used with CPB. When the laceration is in the middle of the posterior left ventricle, external repair can be attempted first. Repair using large interrupted mattress sutures should not be attempted as the myocardium is fragile and will not be able to hold tension while the heart is full and beating.

44 Whenever dealing with a pregnant trauma patient, the focus of resuscitation is on the mother. In a stable patient, who has a viable fetus documented by ultrasound, there are a number of possible approaches. It should be remembered that because of the posterolateral incision needed for repair of the aortic injury, there will be no chance to perform Caesarean section. Caesarean before operation has been described, but delivering a 24-week-old neonate is obviously not desirable. Another approach is to perform the repair using a heparin-bonded (e.g. Biomedicus) atrial to femoral by-pass, keeping distal mean perfusion pressures above 60 mmHg (8.0 kPa). Following repair, premature labour can be arrested with tocolytics. When the child is at full term, as long as blood pressure is controlled, there should be no problem with vaginal delivery.

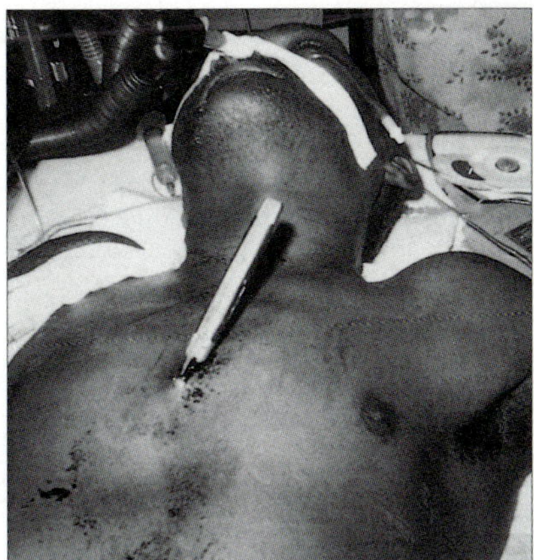

45a

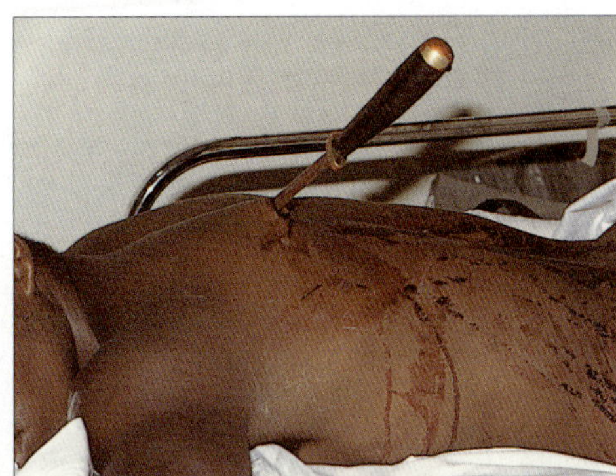

45b

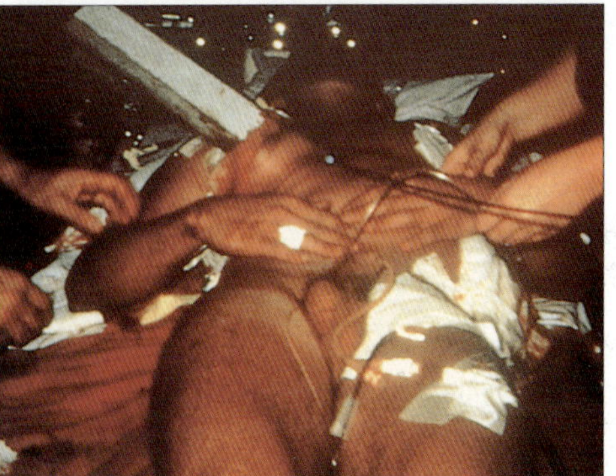

45c

45 What is the common factor in managing these patients (**45a–c**)?

46 A 55-year-old man is on the OR table awaiting urgent coronary bypass. He has severe four vessel coronary disease and unstable angina. Despite sedation and IV nitroglycerine, he complains of chest pain and ECG shows 3.0 mm ST elevation in his anterolateral leads. Discuss the managment of this patient.

47 What are the Class II antidysrhythmics?

48 What is the 'calcium paradox'?

45 All three of these patients have retained objects in their chest. ATLS principles should be used initially. The objects should not be pulled out except in the OR. Patients with objects in the back may have to be intubated while lying between the OR table and stretcher. Most surgeons would perform exploration without removing the object, although occasionally it may be possible to remove the knife etc. after the patient is asleep and then determine whether sternotomy or thoracotomy is needed.

46 The approach includes reassurance and attempts to alleviate the patient's anxiety. Clinical assessment includes looking for signs of pallor and shortness of breath. The administration of oxygen and IV narcotics should be started. Nitroglycerine should be cautiously started if not already being given, taking care to avoid hypotension. If symptoms are associated with significant bradycardia, a pacing pulmonary catheter should be considered. It should be noted that the placement of the patient in a Trendelenburg position may actually make the situation worse as it increases preload and, therefore, myocardial oxygen demand, not to mention aggravating pulmonary oedema. If there is evidence of ongoing ischaemia, intra-aortic balloon counter pulsation should be instituted as soon as possible. Inotropic agents should be used as a last resort, only if there is evidence of cardiogenic shock. Rapid institution of CPB is required whilst the outlined medical efforts are continued; prolonged delay is hazardous. The use of internal mammary grafts is relatively contraindicated in this situation.

47 Class II agents include beta-blockers, which prolong AV node conduction and depress automaticity. They can be used to treat patients with prolonged QT interval, with torsades, supraventricular and ventricular arrhythmias. Cardioselective beta-blockers have more β_1 effects and may reduce the incidence of ventricular fibrillation following MI and cardiac surgery. However, significant side effects include aggravating heart failure, heart block and aggravating asthma or COPD. Shorter acting forms, esmolol and labetolol, are useful also to control undesirable sinus tachycardia and hypertension in patients with aortic dissection or aneurysms. Because of their shorter half-life, better control can be maintained.

48 Intracellular calcium plays a major role in the pathophysiology of reperfusion injury. Reducing calcium during cardioplegic arrest does appear to improve post pump cardiac function. However, cardioplegic arrest with calcium-free solutions is associated with a severe reperfusion injury when re-exposed to calcium. This 'calcium paradox' has been linked to avid calcium uptake, and indeed small amounts of calcium are important for the maintenance of cellular integrity.

49 A 75-year-old man is admitted to the ICU with acute onset of respiratory distress. His past medical history is unremarkable. His chest radiograph is clear and a pulmonary angiogram is performed (**49**). Pulmonary embolism is diagnosed and thrombolysis is considered. Accepted thrombolytic regimens include:

i. Streptokinase 250,000 IU over 30 min followed by an infusion of 100,000 IU/h for 24 h.

ii. Urokinase 4400 IU/kg over 10 min followed by 4400 IU/kg/h for 12 h.

iii. rt-PA 100 mg over 2 h.

iv. All of the above.

v. None of the above.

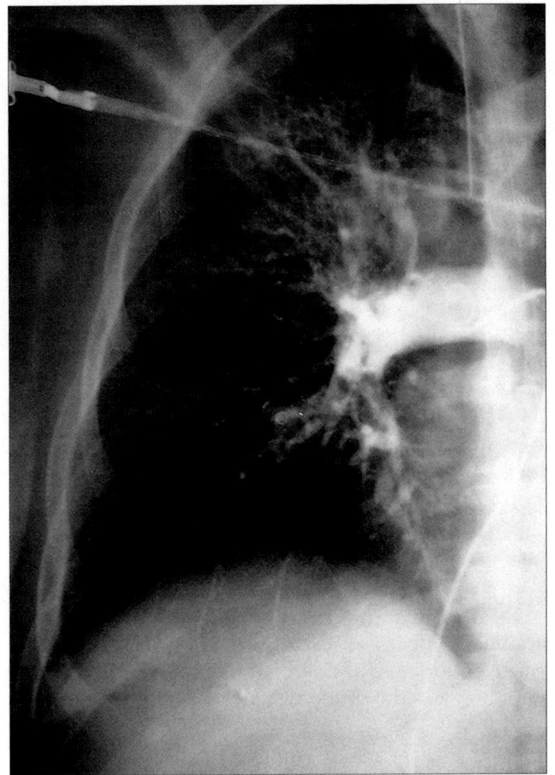

50 An 83-year-old man underwent an uneventful mitral valve replacement. Postoperatively, he was doing well but had persistently low haemoglobin and 2 units of packed red blood cells were transfused. The patient became acutely hypotensive, tachycardic and suffered increasing airways pressure. A rash developed while urine output decreased and became reddish in colour. Shortly thereafter, purpuric lesions were noted, as was increased bleeding from the chest tube. Discuss your approach to this patient.

51 A reduction of diameter of a tube by 50% results in what reduction in cross-sectional area? A reduction in diameter by 75% results in what reduction of cross-sectional area?

52 Discuss selective decontamination of the gut in ventilated patients.

49 iv. Streptokinase, urokinase and rt-PA are thrombolytic agents that are used in fixed or weight-adjusted doses. No laboratory tests are needed during the thrombolytic infusion since no dosage adjustments are made. Heparin is not used concomitantly. A heparin infusion (without loading dose) is started when the PTT is less than 80 s.

50 This patient appears to have had a haemolytic transfusion reaction having developed hypotension, tachycardia, haemoglobinuria and DIC. Additionally, the difficulty in airway ventilation may be due to bronchospasm. Such a severe reaction implies ABO mismatch. Mortality can be as high as 20%. Management includes immediately stopping the transfusion, administering 100% oxygen, increasing intravascular volume, and the administration of adrenaline (0.02–0.05 mg/kg/min). A blood sample should be checked for potential DIC as well as redoing the cross-match. The urine flow should be augmented with volume expansion and osmotic diuretics as initial management.

51 Cross-sectional area = πr^2. A 50% reduction in diameter leads to a 75% reduction in cross-sectional area. A 75% reduction in diameter results in approximately 95% reduction in cross-sectional area. When considering angiography, it is important to recall that the 'normal' vessel which is used to determine the extent of narrowing may itself be diffusely narrowed.

52 The basic concepts on which selective gut decontamination is based are:

- Nosocomial infections are a common problem in the ICU.
- These infections directly contribute to mortality.
- A majority of the infections are due to Gram negative aerobic bacteria that have colonized the oral pharynx from the bowel.

The goals of gut decontamination then are to decrease the colonization rate of these high-risk patients, thereby reducing the incidence of infections and hence improving survival.

Two recent reviews have demonstrated that selective gut decontamination can definitely prevent colonization of the oro-pharynx and intestine with Gram negative aerobic bacteria. The rate of infections was also demonstrated to be reduced by at least 50%. However, the clinical emphasis of gut decontamination in these high-risk ventilated patients remains controversial since both studies did not demonstrate an improvement in survival.

Most selective gut decontamination regimens have three components:

- An oral pharyngeal component with a paste that is applied.
- A gastric component of antibiotics and anti-fungal agents that are given PO.
- A systemic component that includes some sort of IV antibiotic.

53 During a routine coronary bypass, you notice that a bolus of air has just entered through the aortic cannula. Discuss the immediate management and expected outcome.

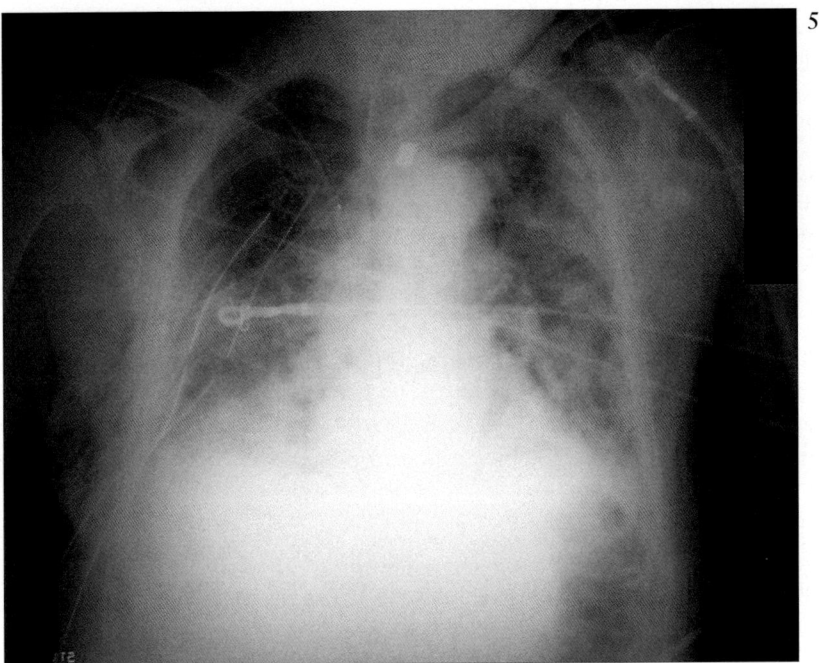

54

54 This patient, admitted because of aspiration and subsequent development of ARDS, is started on Nipride because of systemic hypertension. He subsequently becomes hypoxic with evidence of increased shunt. What is the possible pharmacological basis for this phenomenon?

55 i. Which is the most common cause of syncopal episodes, bradycardia or tachycardia?
ii. What do the five letters that describe a pacemaker represent?
iii. What is physiological pacing?

53 The incidence of air embolism during CPB is very rare, at approximately 0.003% of cases. Causes include: air introduced during cardioplegia administration; inadvertent lowering of the venous reservoir level so that air is 'sucked' into the pump (BOs); retained air during open heart procedures; excessive suction on a vent which pulls air into a chamber; rupture of arterial pumphead tubing; miscellaneous other causes.

When massive air embolism is recognized, the following steps should be performed:

- Stop the pump.
- Place the patient in the Trendelenburg position.
- Vent the aorta.
- Cannulate the SVC for retrograde perfusion.
- 100% oxygen.
- Massage the heart to clear the coronaries.
- Clamp CAB grafts to minimize coronary air.
- Cool the patient to achieve profound hypothermia, usually for 30 min.
- Consider steroids and thiopentone (although this is not proven).
- Simultaneously, find the cause.
- In the last 30 s of retrograde perfusion, have the anaesthesiologist apply carotid pressure (to flush the vertebrals).

The outcome is grim and probably 25–50% mortality can be expected. The use of thiopentone may delay an appreciation of the severity of neurological deficit for 2–3 days.

54 Hypoxic pulmonary vasoconstriction is one 'defence' mechanism that may reduce shunting. Blocking this with a vasodilator, such as Nipride or nitroglycerine, may increase shunt as in this case. Prolonged use of Nipride, particularly if there is renal dysfunction, can result in thiocyanate toxicity also leading to 'increased shunt'. This is associated with tinnitus, blurred vision and delirium. At increasing levels, cyanide intoxication can occur, with inability of the cells to take up oxygen. This leads to an 'oxygen saturation gap' in which there is a >5% difference between measured and calculated saturation. Additionally, lactic acidosis will occur. Treatment of this potentially fatal complication is the administration of amyl nitrate inhalations and IV sodium thiosulphate.

55 i. Syncopal episodes are due to bradycardic events in 85% of cases, tachyarrhythmias in 15%.
ii The first letter refers to the chamber paced (V, A, D = dual), the second to the chamber sensed (V, A, D, O = none), and the third letter to the mode (I = inhibited, T = triggered, D = double, O = none). The fourth letter refers to programmable modes (R = rate responsive, etc), and the fifth letter to special functions (B = burst, S = scanning, etc).
iii. Physiological pacing can refer to synchronized AV pacing, such as with DDD or it can refer to pacemakers that are programmed to respond to body activity, temperature, pH, etc, to increase with activity or stress.

56 Which point in the graph (56) represents the state of maximal potential tension development and why?

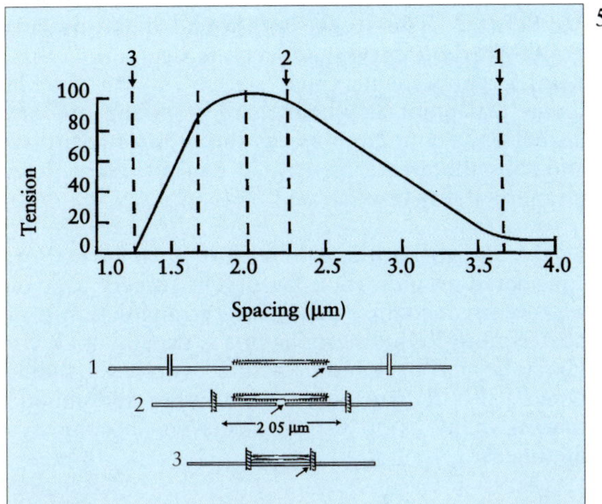

57 The patient with this radiograph (57) is best treated by:
i. Gastroscopy and conservative treatment.
ii. Urgent surgery.
iii. Elective surgery in all cases.
iv. Elective surgery for symptomatic cases only.
v. Elective surgery for cases only with reflux oesophagitis.

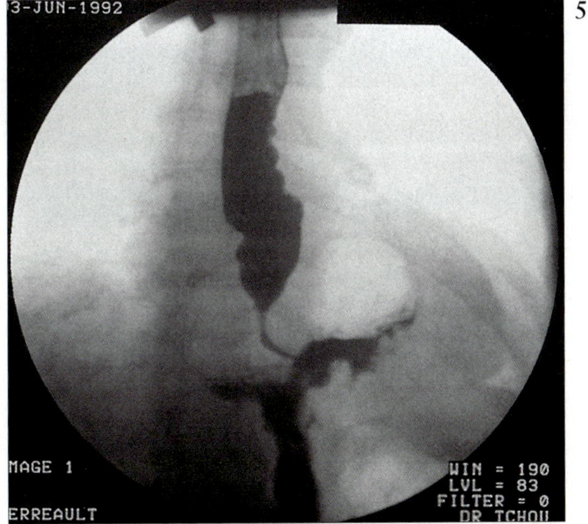

58 Ten minutes after the institution of CPB, the anaesthesiologist and the surgeons simultaneously note that the blood arterial inflow line is very dark. Blood gas sampling of the arterial profusion line reveals a PaO_2 of 50 mmHg (6.6 kPa). What are the causes of this problem?

59 Discuss ulcer prophylaxis in the ventilated ICU patient.

56 Point 2. The stroke work–end diastolic relationship (such as described by Frank–Starling curves) reflect the degree of cross bridging between the filaments. Point 1 represents maximal 'stretch', so that the filaments cannot interact. This is the theoretical point at which there is 'falling off' of the Starling curve with excessive distention. Point 2 represents the most efficient overlap of thick and thin filaments, and thus the greater generated tension. Point 3 represents maximal crowding, with no more ability to contract.

57 iv. Paraoesophageal hernias with intrathoracic stomachs were in the past considered an indication for urgent surgery to avoid gastric strangulation. However, we recently recognize that gastric strangulation is rare except in symptomatic cases of obstruction. Reflux oesophagitis is usually not a common symptom with this disease. Hiatal hernias have been classified as types I (sliding only), II (paraoesophageal only), type III (I + II) and type IV (i.e. other abdominal structures involved). Having said this, as many as 50% of patients will become symptomatic at some point in their lifetime.

58 Causes can be due to a malfunction of the gas supply system or the oxygenator. Immediate arterial blood gas analysis must be made and the perfusionist should simultaneously increase O_2 gas flows and check the mechanical pump flow. An inspection of all the gases and tubing should be made as well as an inspection of the oxygenator to ensure appropriate blood levels. Arterial and venous lines should be checked by the surgeons to make sure of all appropriate connections. If CPB has been instituted prior to cardiac arrest, consideration should be given to allowing the heart to continue to beat while continuing to ventilate the lungs. Such oxygen delivery problems are more common with the BOs rather than the more current MOs.

59 Stress ulcers occur in patients following severe burn trauma, haemorrhagic shock, respiratory failure or sepsis. They consist of multiple superficial erosions that occur primarily in the fundus of the stomach. These erosions are clearly different from Cushing's ulcer, ulcers induced by drugs and re-activation of a pre-existing chronic ulcer. The latter may often perforate as they are frequently a full thickness ulceration. The pathway in the development of stress ulceration is the reduced ability of the stomach to protect itself against acid injury due to back diffusion of acid rather than increased amounts of acid secretion. Low flow and/or sepsis contribute to ischaemia of the gastric mucosa. The role of bile reflux as well as *H. pylori* is felt to be less significant in causing stress ulceration.
  Prophylaxis revolves around attempts to reduce gastric acidity and has been shown in a number of prospective trials to prevent severe upper GI bleeding in critically ill ventilated patients. Many authors advocate the use of either antacids or H_2 blockers to neutralize gastric acid. However, recently there has been increased enthusiasm for the use of sucralfate as it does not change the gastric pH and may result in reduced nosocomial pneumonia in these patients. Omeprazole is used for established peptic ulceration in high-risk patients.

60 What are the Class IA antidysrhythmics?

61 This is a representation of the ECG 'vectors' in horizontal plane (61). What leads do the 0, −30, −150, 120, 90, 60 vectors correlate with?

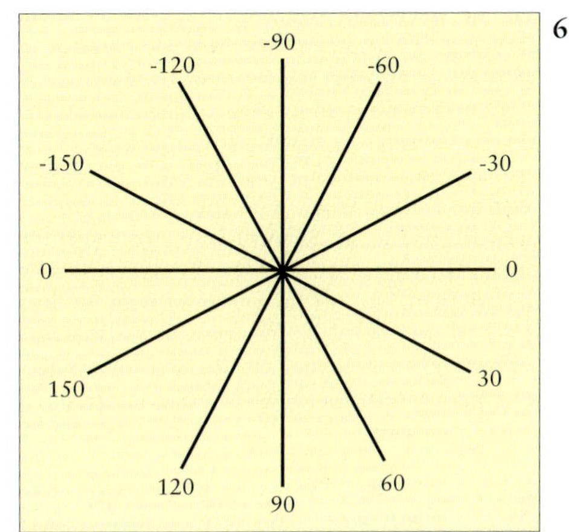

62 This chest radiograph is that of a 24-year-old woman who has been transported to the trauma room following a RTA (62). The patient is hypotensive with a blood pressure of 90/60 mmHg (12.0/8.0 kPa) and a pulse of 130 b.p.m. The accident was described as a high-energy impact/head-on collision and the patient was entrapped by her lower extremities for approximately 20 min. There are obvious significant orthopaedic injuries including a mid-shaft femur fracture and bilateral open tibial fractures. The patient fails to stabilize after 2 l of crystalloid infusion, the application of MAST trousers and 9 units of red cell concentrate. A diagnostic peritoneal lavage is clear or colourless. Subsequent evaluation reveals a significant intrathoracic process. What is your differential diagnosis and what confirmatory diagnostic approach(es) might be considered?

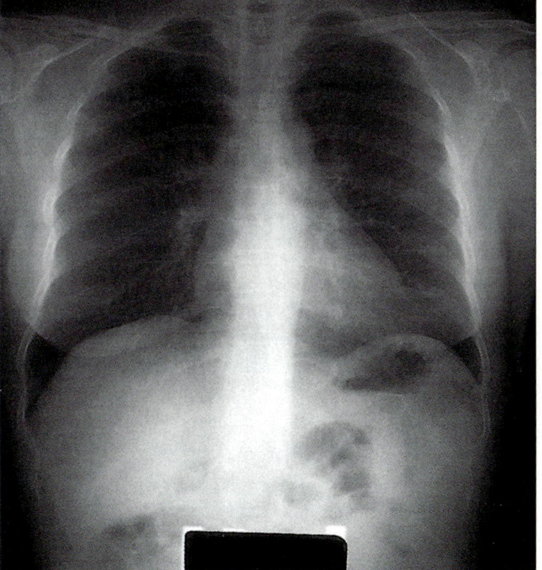

60 Class I, the local anaesthetics, have been divided into three subsets. Class IA includes quinidine, procainamide and dysopyramide. These have the effect of depressing phase 0, decreasing conduction velocity and prolonging phase 4. All three can be used for supraventricular as well as ventricular dysrhythmias. All three can prolong QT interval and induce torsades. They should not be given for wide complex tachyarrhythmias, therefore, unless one is sure that the arrhythmia is not ventricular. Procainamide is metabolized to an active breakdown product, NAPA. When drawing levels, therefore, both procaine and NAPA levels can be followed. The QRS should also be monitored. If the length increases greater than 50%, procainamide should be withheld. Side effects include hypotension, drowsiness, myalgia and Raynaud's. Both procainamide and quinidine are useful in treating supraventricular and ventricular arrhythmias. Side effects attributed to quinidine which include myocardial depression, vasodilation resulting in hypotension, allergic reactions, GI upset and mild to severe CNS effects. Quinidine results in increased digoxin levels, necessitating adjustment of dosing. It should be noted that, as a rule, drug levels of both quinidine and procainamide/NAPA do not appear to correlate well with efficacy or predicting complications.

61 0 = I; –30 = aVL; –150 = aVR; 120 = III; 90 = aVF; 60 = II. Normal axis is between +90 and –30. –30 to –90 = LAD. –90 to 180 = marked RAD. 180 to +90 = RAD.

62 The patient has sustained a blunt rupture of the right atrium with resultant cardiac tamponade. The radiograph demonstrates normal thoracic landmarks without evidence of tension pneumothorax, pneumothorax or haemothorax. The pericardial silhouette is unremarkable. The tough and fibrous pericardium does not accommodate acutely and significant haemodynamic compromise can occur in patients with a radiographically normal cardiac silhouette. The diagnosis of cardiac injury with tamponade should be considered in the patient who has suffered significant blunt force trauma and fails to respond to standard resuscitation measures. Concomitant intra-abdominal haemorrhage, orthopaedic and neurologic injuries must be rapidly assessed and addressed. Clinical signs associated with cardiac tamponade include muffled heart sounds, jugular venous distention, and hypotension (Beck's triad). The placement of a CVP monitoring line may distinguish this entity from other traumatic aetiologies. In the setting of cardiac tamponade the CVP may be expected to be elevated in contradistinction to traumatic hypovolaemic haemorrhagic shock. (Echocardiogram is the most reliable test for detecting pericardial fluid, as an important differential diagnosis is 'myocardial contusion'.) Aggressive volume resuscitation may be required, particularly in the face of associated injuries. Pericardiocentesis may provide transient improvement but should not delay preparation and transport to the OR.

63 The flow–volume loop on the left is normal (63). What does the one on the right demonstrate?

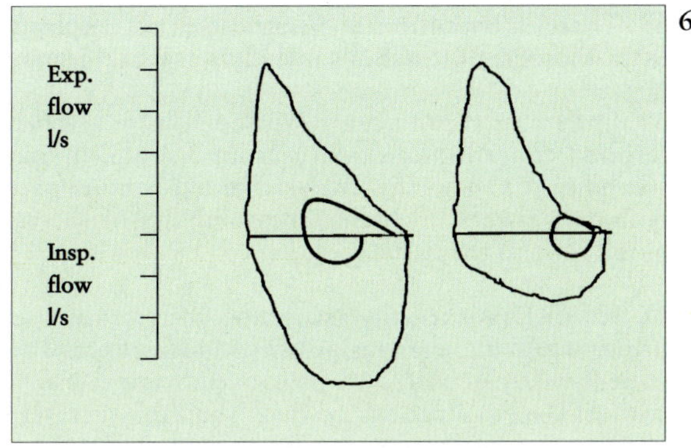

64 Discuss factors governing the uptake and distribution of inhalational agents.

65 A 50-year-old white man is unconscious and ventilator-dependent 5 days after subarachnoid haemorrhage secondary to hypertensive crisis. The blood pressure is 120/80 mmHg (16.0–10.7 kPa), pulse is 90 b.p.m., respirations are 20 breaths/min and temperature is 38°C. He is producing adequate urine and has a CVP of 8 mmHg (1.1 kPa).

His blood pressure drops to 80/60 mmHg (10.7–8.0 kPa), heart rate is 120 b.p.m., CVP and urine output are unchanged. Systolic blood pressure rises to only 100 mmHg (13.3 kPa) despite 10 µg/kg/min of dopamine.

The following laboratory values are obtained: sodium is 132 mmol/l (132 mEq/l), potassium is 4.0 mmol/l (4.0 mEq/l), chloride and bicarbonate are normal. Urine sodium is 30 mmol/l (30 mEq/l), osmolality is 290 mosm. Serum cortisol is drawn on this patient and it is 18 mg/dl (1.8 mg/ml). The diagnosis of this patient would include the following possibilities:

i. Diabetes insipidus.
ii. SIADH.
iii. Cerebral salt wasting syndrome.
iv. Adrenal insufficiency.

63 There is limitation of inspiration, not expiration. This can be seen with fixed extra-thoracic obstructions including tracheal tumours or tracheomalacia.

64 Important factors can be grouped into: alveolar partial pressure, determined by inspired concentration and ventilation rate; uptake from lungs which is related to solubility, CO and the alveolar-mixed venous partial pressure gradient; and distribution of tissues, including the solubility of the agents in the tissues as well as the blood flow to the tissue.

65 iv. SIADH is usually associated with a lower serum osmolality and concentrated urine, while diabetes insipidus produces excessive urine. The urinary sodium in a patient with cerebral salt wasting syndrome is usually much higher than listed. Serum cortisol level in a patient in shock should be greater than 20 mg/dl (2 mg/ml).

Adrenal insufficiency can be either be primary or secondary. The primary causes are:

- 70% have autoimmune-mediated endocrinopathy that results in adrenal gland destruction;
- destruction of the gland secondary to *Mycobacterium tuberculosis*.

Other causes of primary adrenal insufficiency include bilateral haemorrhagic destruction of the gland secondary to bacterial infection, shock and systemic diseases such as sarcoidosis, malignancy, anaphylaxis or perhaps systemic fungal infection. Secondary adrenal insufficiency may be due to withdrawal of hydrocortisone or other group of corticoid medications, biliary infection, carcinoma, and basilar skull fractures. Patients with loss of mineralocorticoid effect will frequently have hyponatraemia, hyperkalaemia, decreased bicarbonate levels and elevated BUN. They also may have hypoglycaemia.

Diagnosis of adrenal insufficiency in the intensive care unit can be made by a short ACTH stimulation test or what it is commonly referred to as a corticotrophin stimulation test.

Serum samples are obtained just prior to 30 and 60 min after an IV injection of 150 mg of synthetic ACTH (corticotrophin). A normal response is defined as an increase in the cortisol level of at least 7 mg/dl (0.7 mg/ml) over the basal level and a rise in serum cortisol with an absolute level of at least 20 mg/dl (2 mg/ml). Both conditions must be met for a normal response. If this has not occurred, then the test is considered positive and the patient is felt to have adrenal insufficiency. This test does not, however, differentiate between primary and secondary adrenal insufficiency.

66 A 56-year-old patient with a calcific aortic stenosis presents with syncope. Aetiology of syncope is related to:
i. Associated cerebrovascular malformations.
ii. Occurrence of ventricular arrhythmias.
iii. Hyperinsulinaemia.
iv. Decreased cerebral perfusion.

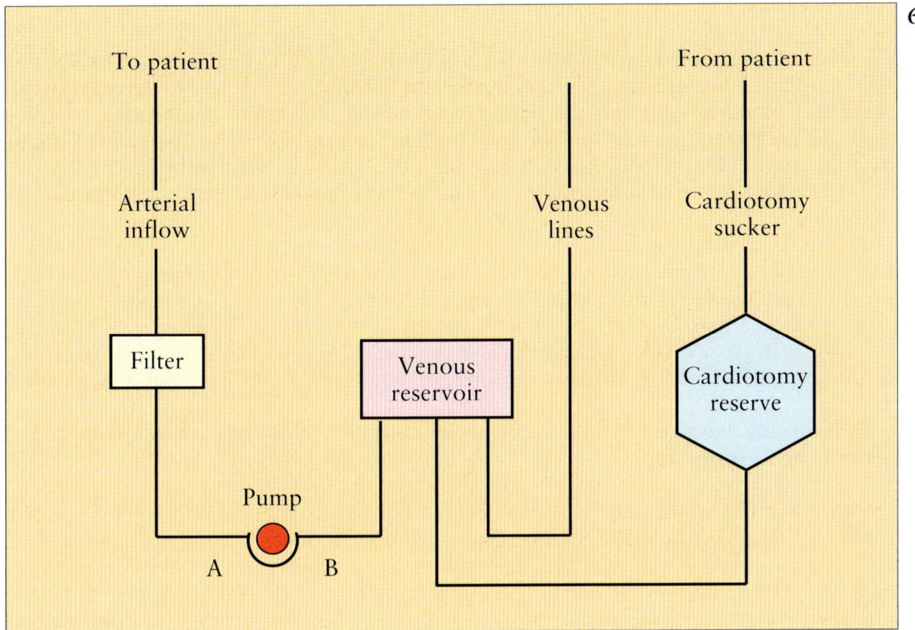

67 In (67) indicate where a MO and a BO would be placed. Describe the advantages and disadvantages of each.

68 Discuss the advantages of the use of fentanyl compared to morphine as a narcotic agent in cardiac patients.

69 Which carries a graver prognosis after acute MI, Mobilitz type I or II block?

66 ii and **iv.** The effort syncope of aortic stenosis is due to decreased cerebral perfusion. The latter is due to decreased CO and/or ventricular arrhythmias. Survival has been estimated at 3–4 years with syncope due to aortic stenosis. Proposed mechanism for syncope is left ventricular failure with an abrupt fall in CO. Ventricular arrhythmias may also contribute to syncope and occur in late stages of circulatory impairment. Exercise-induced peripheral vasodilatation may also aggravate systolic pressure gradient and further reduce perfusion pressure of the myocardium. In older patients with calcific aortic stenosis, transient cerebral ischaemia may also occur secondary to underlying cerebral vascular disease.

67 BOs can be placed proximal to the pump (B). Gas flow determines both O_2 and CO_2 content. They are cheaper and quicker to set up than MOs. However, because there is a blood–gas interface, a defoamer is needed and there is increased complement, leucocyte and platelet activation. This has been correlated with increased organ dysfunction following CPB. Also, there is an increased risk of air emboli (A).

With a MO, gas exchange occurs at a membrane–gas interface. O_2 content can be manipulated independent of gas flow. There is much less blood trauma and subsequently decreased incidence of organ dysfunction compared to BO. There is also a reduced risk of air embolism. MO must be placed downstream of the pump as high pressures are needed to push blood through the device.

68 Morphine can result in significant hypotension, mechanisms for which include histamine release leading to vasodilation and venous pooling. Fentanyl is associated with much less histamine release and is thus the agent of choice for treating patients with poor CO. However, it may be associated with muscular rigidity following emergence from anaesthesia.

69 Moblitz II second degree AV block is characterized by a relatively fixed PR interval, and often the QRS is wide. There are nonconducted beats. In the setting of acute MI, especially anterior MI, this rhythm has a more serious implication than Moblitz type I, because it implies more destruction of the myocardium and conduction system. Atropine and isoproteronol may be helpful transiently, but artificial pacing is usually required.

Moblitz type I (Wenkebach) may exist as a transient phenomenon following MI, and usually does not require pacing. It is characterized by an increasing PR and decreasing RR interval until a beat is dropped (e.g. 3:4 or 2:3). It is more responsive to atropine and isoproteronol than type II block.

In general, heart block following inferior MI is felt to be of lesser significance than following anterior MI as block with anterior MI implies extensive myocardial necrosis and damage.

70 What is wrong with this chest radiograph (**70**) (taken after a line change) and what should be done?

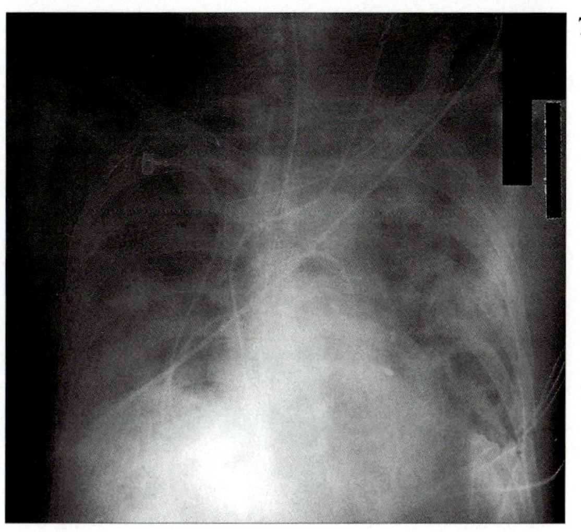

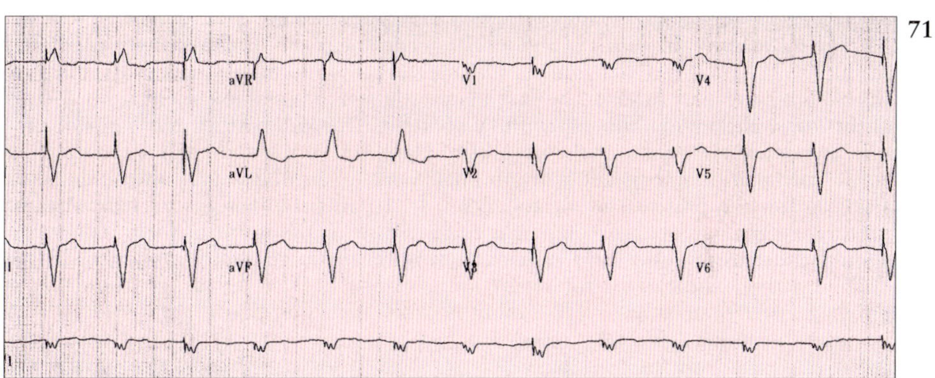

71 **i.** What is the mechanism of the rhythm in this ECG (**71**)?
ii. What would be seen on a portable chest radiograph?

72 What are Class IB antidysrythmics?

73 A 60-year-old man with a history of hypertension and COPD presents to the emergency department with acute epigastric abdominal pain and distention. The pain is constant with radiation to both groins. He is distended without rebound and has a large pulsatile mass in the mid-abdomen. What is the most likely diagnosis and how would this be best confirmed?

70 There is an intravascular guide wire. This illustrates the importance of always holding on to the wire during manipulations. The wire should be removed by the interventional radiologists.

71 i. Electronic ventricular pacemaker. Note the spike before each QRS complex. The complexes are inverted in leads II, III and a VF suggesting a 'bottom-to-top' direction of depolarization of the heart and upright in lead I suggesting a 'right-to-left' direction of depolarization.
ii. These are all consistent with appropriate lead placement in the RV apex, which should be confirmed by a chest radiograph.

72 Class IB agents include lidocaine (lignocaine), phenytoin, tocainamide and mexiletine. These agents are associated with augmented AV node conduction and shortening of phase 4, and have little effect on atrial dysrhythmias. While the use of lidocaine (lignocaine) does appear to reduce the incidence of ventricular arrhythmias following MI and post coronary bypass, the therapeutic ratio has recently been questioned. Lidocaine (lignocaine) is associated with pro-arrhythmic effects, myocardial depression and CNS side effects including seizures. The incidence of side effects is greater in the presence of CHF. Phenytoin is usually used only to treat digoxin-induced arrhythmias. Infusion rates should be less than 50 mg/min to avoid cardiovascular collapse.

73 The most likely diagnosis is abdominal aortic aneurysm, probably with contained rupture. The differential diagnosis includes other abdominal aneurysms, such as splenic artery or iliac artery. The best diagnostic test in a stable patient is a CT scan of the lower chest and abdomen with IV contrast. This will best identify signs of rupture and define the extent of the aneurysm. Plain film of the abdomen demonstrating aortic calcification consistent with an aneurysm, or an abdominal ultrasound may also confirm the presence of an aneurysm. In a patient with signs or symptoms of rupture, emergency operative repair is indicated. It is important in these patients to avoid hypertension, and limit resuscitation until aortic control is obtained. In the elective patient, indications for repair are generally defined as an aneurysm that is growing faster than 5 mm every 6 months or an aneurysm that is greater than 5 cm in antero-posterior diameter.

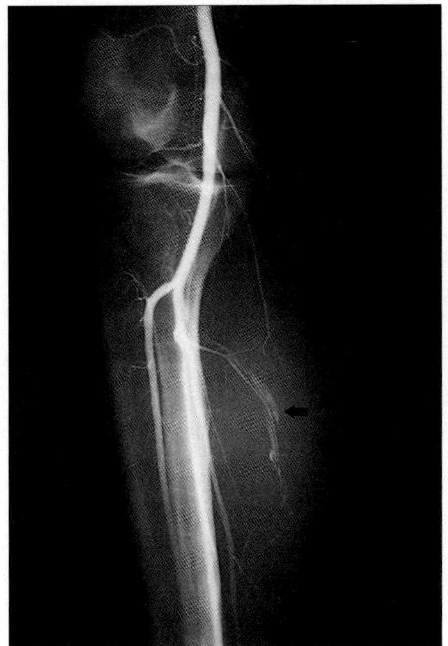

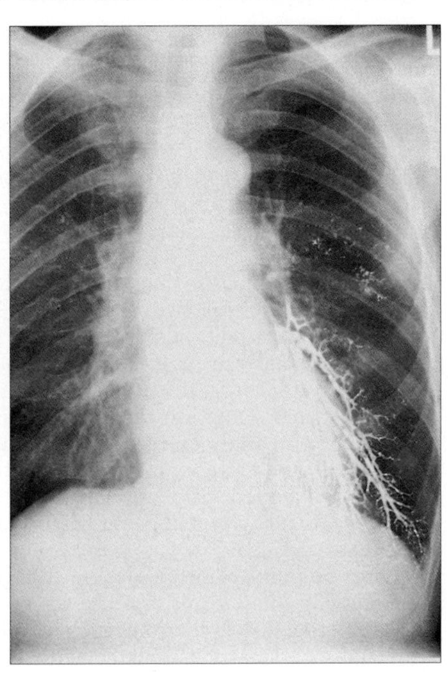

74 A 34-year-old patient presents with a gunshot wound to the right lower extremity. He has a history of IV drug use, with deep venous thrombosis. Examination reveals calf swelling, some loss of sensation in the first web space dorsally and superficial venous distension with a thrill. An angiogram reveals a small AV fistula (74). Discuss indications for surgery in this setting.

75 The best management for a patient with the chest radiograph following a barium swallow and a known history of oesophageal cancer (75) is:
i. NPO IV fluids and antibiotics.
ii. G-tube insertion.
iii. Oesophageal stent insertion.
iv. Bronchus stent insertion.
v. Radiation treatment.

76 What is 'phase II' block?

77 What is WPW syndrome?

74 The patient has evidence of compartment syndrome, and this is the primary indication for surgery. The majority of traumatic AV fistulas will seal spontaneously. They can also be embolized. However, this patient already has deep venous thrombosis and evidence of superficial venous hypertension. Thus, decompression of the calf compartments as well as ligation of the fistula is appropriate in this case.

The commonest cause of compartment syndrome in cardiothoracic surgery is placement of IABP in the femoral artery in patients with low CO and/or aortoiliac occlusive disease. This clinical scenario is rare in the UK.

75 **iii.** This patient has barium in the left borders, consistent with oesophageal-bronchial or tracheal fistula. Despite the morbidity with an oesophageal stent because of aspiration, a well-placed stent will occlude the fistula and prevent further contamination of the lung and allow the patient to swallow again. IV fluids and gastrostomy tubes do not address the major morbidity here which is continuing pulmonary contamination through the fistula. Radiation treatment is still debated and has the potential of enlarging the fistula. A bronchus stent should be of use only if combined with an oesophageal stent and if there was a bronchiostenosis which was preventing adequate bronchus drainage. (Even with timely intervention, the prognosis for patients with malignant tracheoesophageal fistulas remains poor.)

76 Large amounts of succinylcholine, a depolarizing muscle relaxant (usually greater than 5 mg/kg) may result in a change in the nature of the neuromuscular blockade. While post-synaptic membrane becomes repolarized, it becomes insensitive to acetylcholine. This is associated with tetanic fade and decreased response on the fourth compared to the first twitch (less than 70%) in the train of four. The duration of this phase II desensitization ('phase II' block) varies and there is only limited success with neostigmine. Generally, treatment is supportive, including ventilation until the block resolves.

77 WPW syndrome is a form of AV nodal re-entrant tachyarrhythmia, or pre-excitation arrhythmia. In orthodromic pattern, a normal impulse is conducted antegrade via the AV node but retrograde via the accessory pathway between the atria and ventricle. In antidromic form, the reverse is true. The pre-excitation of the ventricle produces a shorter PR interval (<120 ms), a 'delta' wave, which is a slurring of the initial QRS (a fusion complex) and this in turn results in a wider QRS (>20 ms).

78 A 67-year-old woman was admitted to the respiratory ICU with pneumonia requiring ventilatory support. She progressively deteriorates with evidence of confusion and develops hypothermia. Upon attempts to wean the patient from the ventilator, she develops hypercarbia. Her past history indicates that heart failure and stroke might occur. Examination reveals a scar on the patient's neck and her family say that she may have had a thyroidectomy. Discuss the management of this patient.

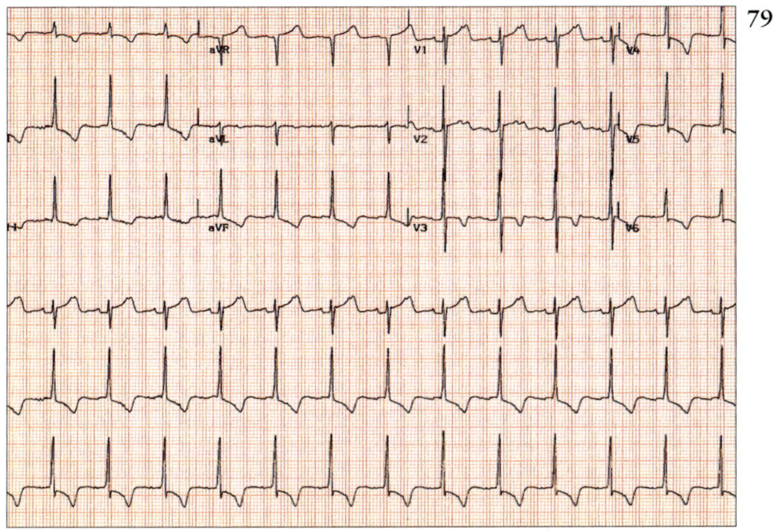

79 What abnormalities are present on this ECG?

80 A patient presented with complaints of shortness of breath for the past two weeks. He had had a prior pneumothorax treated with tube drainage. His chest radiograph is shown (80). Shortly after performing tube thoracostomy, and placing the tube to suction, he develops dyspnoea, cyanosis and frothy pulmonary secretions. Discuss the prevention and management of this complication.

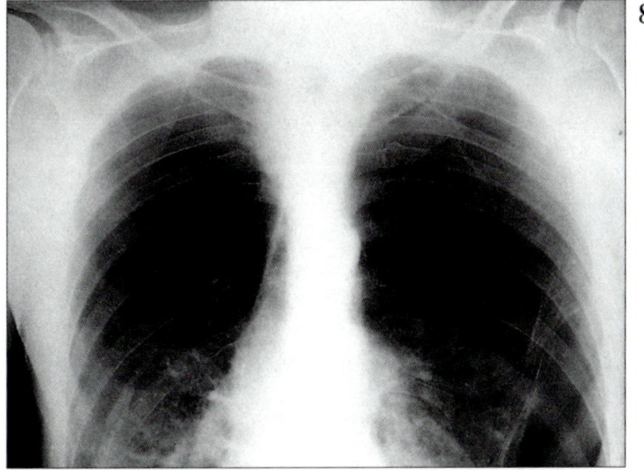

78 This patient may very well have myxoedema. Myxoedema is more commonly seen in elderly patients and is often precipitated by pulmonary infections. Other triggering factors include: the use of barbiturates; respiratory failure; CHF; CVA; trauma; cold exposure; GI haemorrhage; hypoglycaemia; hyponatraemia; hypo-adrenalism; surgery and seizures. Evaluation includes measurement of serum TSH and T_4 levels. Treatment involves warming, treatment with IV fluids, hydrocortisone 100 mg IV every 8 h, and IV L-thyroxine (LT_4). The dose of IV LT_4 has been recommended from 100 mg daily up to a bolus of 500 mg followed by 100 mg daily. Some authors recommend 25 mg of T_3 every 6 h as severely hypothyroid patients may have a blocked version of T_4 to T_3. Respiratory failure may be related to decreased CNS response to hypoxic and hypercarbic drives and/or weakened respiratory muscles. Contributing factors need to be treated.

79 There is ST depression inferiorly and ST changes in the anterolateral leads, consistent with ischaemia. When ST segments are depressed, the ischaemia may be reversible. ST elevation implies some degree of myocardial injury, but if diffuse are consistent with pericarditis. Q waves indicate transmural infarction ('completed' injury).

80 Re-expansion pulmonary oedema is a unilateral oedema that occurs following re-expansion of a chronically collapsed lung, either from effusion or pneumothorax. Negative pleural pressures, associated with chest tube suction, appear to aggravate trans-pleural fluid shifts. Rapid and forceful expansion by positive pressure venti-lation can be a further inciting factor. Prevention includes recognizing the chronicity of the condition (days to weeks). Initially placing the tube thoracostomy to water seal only for a few hours may allow more gentle expansion. If a large effusion is being drained, limiting the amount to 1000 ml initially and then periodically allowing a few 100 ml to drain off can prevent re-expansion oedema. Once it occurs, treatment is largely supportive and can include diuretics, oxygen and mechanical ventilation. The course is usually short, lasting less than 48 h.

81 Seven days following a RTA, a 47-year-old man with a past history of smoking developed a lesion seen on the radiograph. Subsequent CT are shown (**81a, b**). He is entirely asymptomatic. The next step in the management is:
i. Clinical observation.
ii. Serial chest radiograph until it resolves.
iii. Bronchoscopy.
iv. CT guided aspiration and drainage.
v. Surgical resection.

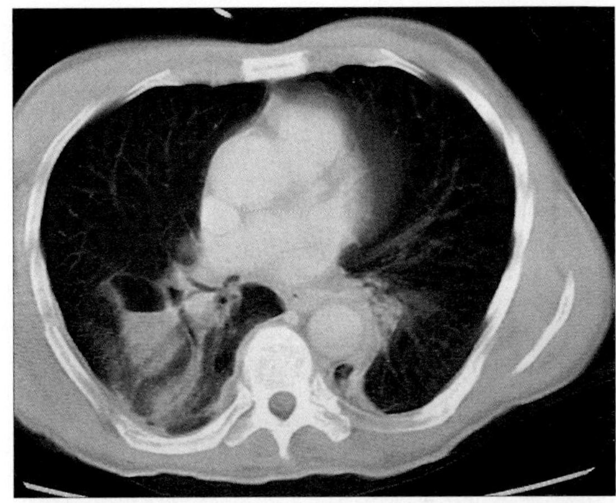

81a

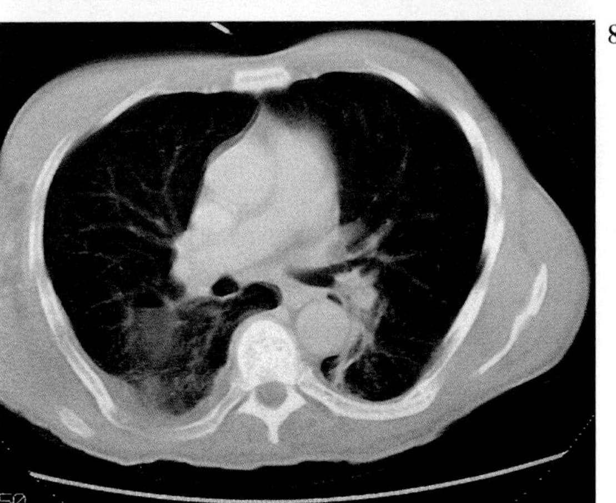

81b

82 A 22-year-old college student is admitted after a suicide attempt during which she ingested a large amount of insecticide. She presents with myoclonic seizures, weakness, salivation and then develops significant respiratory muscle depression. Discuss your treatment.

83 A 72-year old male who suffered a cardiac arrest 6 hours ago is intubated and has a radial arterial line and a Swan–Ganz catheter in place. Discuss two different methods of determining CO in this patient.

81 ii. The lesion illustrated is a pneumatocele. Pneumatoceles may be associated with air–fluid levels, and can occur in a delayed fashion in an area of pulmonary contusion. Complications include infection and rupture. The clinical course is determined by the size of the pneumatocele, presence or absence of complications, and severity of underlying contusion. Uncomplicated pneumatocele tends, on CT, to have sharp clear margins without signs of parenchymal inflammation. While as many as 40% of patients can present with haemoptysis or cough, the majority of patients need only be watched expectantly. Serial CXRs for 1–2 days, to ensure that the lesion is not growing, is all that is required. If there is concern about possible superinfection, radiologically guided aspiration and drainage may be appropriate.

82 Supportive approaches include the treatment of any associated arrhythmias, respiratory support and IV fluids. Atropine is useful for treating seizures, arrhythmias and excessive salivation. Pralidoxine (2 pam) is useful for treating respiratory muscle failure. Dose in the adult is 2 g IV in 250 ml of normal saline over 30 min and in the paediatric population, 25–50 mg/kg is administered in the same fashion. It is most effective when used in the initial 24–36 h after exposure and may be repeated every hour for 8 h.

83 The reverse Fick method and thermodilution method are two ways of determining CO. The reverse Fick equation is used if whole body oxygen consumption can be measure by analysis of inspired oxygen and expired oxygen by indirect calorimetry. Oxygen consumption is then divided by the difference of the arterial and mixed venous oxygen content:

$$CO \text{ (l/min)} = VO_2/(CaO_2art - CaO_2ven)$$

where VO_2 is oxygen consumption (ml/min), CaO_2art (ml/l) is arterial oxygen content and CaO_2ven (ml/l) is central venous oxygen content. This method can only be used in steady state and when no type of right-to-left or left-to-right shunt exists. This is most often used in research models.

The thermodilution method is a common method of determining CO when a Swan–Ganz catheter is in place. A thermistor is at the tip of the Swan–Ganz catheter which is inserted in the PA. CO is determined when a known temperature (4°C) and known amount of saline (10 ml) is injected in the right atrium along with venous blood returning to the heart. The venous blood and cold saline is mixed in the right ventricle where it then flows through the PA and thermistor. The Stewart–Hamilton formula is then used to calculate CO:

$$CO = (V(Tb - T1)\ K1K2)/{^\wedge}Tb(t)dt$$

where V = injected volume, Tb = blood temperature, T_1 = injectate temperature, ${^\wedge}Tb(t)dt$ = change in blood temperature as a function of time and K_1 and K_2 are constants. This method assumes no heat is absorbed from the rest of the body, homogeneous distribution of the injectate in the right ventricle, no left-to-right shunt and no valvular insufficiency.

84 This is a representation of 'normal' and 'septic' relationship between O_2 delivery and consumption (84). Discuss the relative arguments for and against using PAOC-derived data for 'goal-directed therapy'.

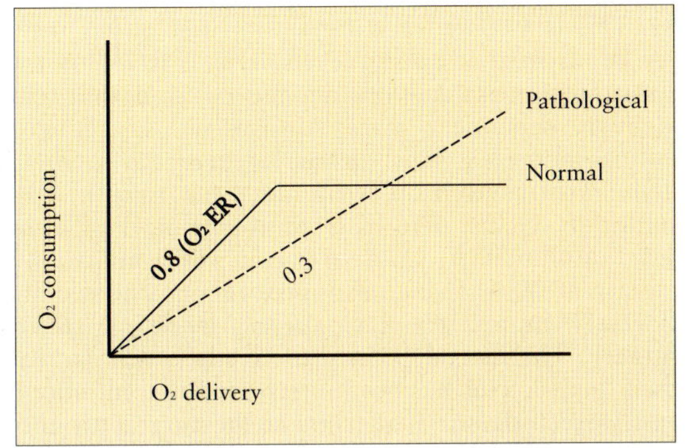

85 An otherwise healthy newborn male, weighing 2.4 kg (born of an uneventful pregnancy and delivery) develops tachypnoea at 48 hours of life. His SaO_2 is 90% in room air and 99% with 3/4 l/min of O_2. There is no evidence of congenital heart disease and an echocardiogram is normal. A chest radiograph was taken (85). The optimal (long-term) management of this condition is:

i. Trocar/cannula decompression of the left chest.
ii. Selective endobronchial intubation.
iii. Rigid bronchoscopy to suction mucus plugs.
iv. ECMO.
v. Thoracotomy and resection of the involved lobe/segment.

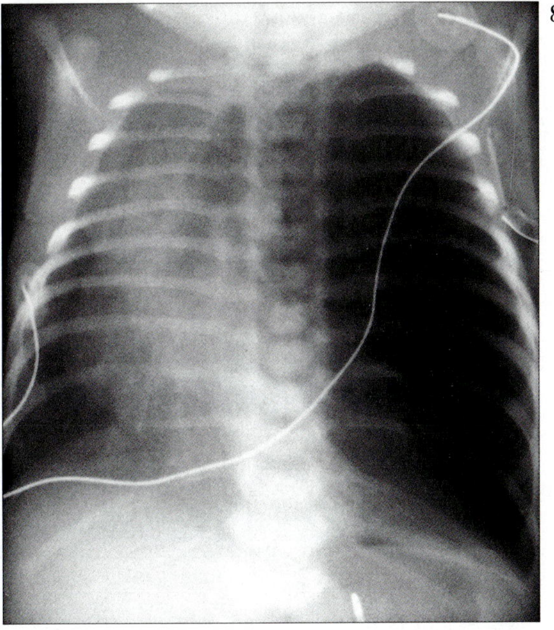

86 What are Class IC antidysrythmics?

84 This is a controversial area. In brief, some investigators feel that CI and O_2 delivery be targeted at certain levels. This is based on the belief that at some point oxygen consumption is 'delivery dependent' and that as long as a patient remains in the 'delivery dependent' state, survival will be reduced and the incidence of end-organ failure increased. It is further argued that in the sepsis syndrome, the slope of O_2 delivery–consumption is blunted, resulting in continuous flow-dependent O_2 consumption. Goals, derived from averaging data from survivors, have included a CI of 4.5 l/min/m² BSA; O_2 delivery of >600 ml/min/m² BSA; O_2 consumption of >170 ml/min/m² BSA. Using vasopressors and dobutamine, this approach has been used in 'severely' injured trauma patients, septic patients and 'patient's at risk' undergoing surgery. The mortality, in some studies, was increased in those patients not reaching their 'goals'. This has been interpreted in a number of ways including disease so severe as to preclude survival (thus suggesting a prognostic value of this approach) and primary cardiac dysfunction on the basis of sepsis.

However, there is not universal acceptance of this approach. Critics note that there is a mathematical 'coupling' of these indices, and further, that if the primary pathophysiology of sepsis and haemorrhagic shock is shunting and closure of capillary beds, in addition to intracellular volume loss, the use of vasopressors may actually aggravate the process. Further, if there is a primary cardiac dysfunction, such an approach may actually result in increased cardiac complications. In addition, independent measurement of O_2 consumption suggests that the perceived 'flow-dependent oxygen consumption' does not really exist. Also, there is evidence to suggest that the use of pressors creates increased oxygen consumption by increasing myocardial demand and thermogenesis ('physiologic coupling'). Additionally, in ARDS, it is also proposed that the primary process leading to 'hypoxia' is in fact shorter capillary transit times, with resultant decreased uptake of O_2 by red blood cells. The transit time would be further decreased by forcing CO to be greater. Finally, even proponents of such 'PAOC' based therapy recognize that in the studies purporting to show benefit, the target goals were not actually met. Clinical studies are contradictory, with some suggesting no harm, some a benefit and some a detrimental effect to 'goal-directed therapy'. Ultimately, this approach must still be validated before widespread usage can be recommended.

85 v. Congenital lobar emphysema is almost always present at birth, becomes rapidly progressive, and usually affects only one lobe, invariably the upper lobe, but in very rare instances may be bilateral. Associated anomalies are uncommon and with progressive distension of the affected lobe, there is mediastinal shift and atelectasis of the ipsilateral lower lobe and ultimately the contralateral lung. As a temporary measure, selective contralateral endobronchial intubation may be used. (Most commonly, this involves intubating the right main stem bronchus to relieve overinflation of the left upper lobe.) Definitive treatment is urgent thoracotomy and resection of the involved lobe/segment. The majority of children present within the first four weeks of life, but occasionally the condition will not be diagnosed until later childhood.

86 Class IC agents include flecainide and encainide. These agents have major impact on phase 0. These agents were tried in a study of long term suppression of ventricular ectopy following MI. Pro-arrhythmic rates of up to 25% were noted with possibly increased mortality. These agents are restricted to resistant malignant ventricular tachyarrhythmias.

87 This 24-year-old man was shot 8 hours ago in the right chest by a rival drug dealer. He had an angiogram (87) at another institution and is now referred to your centre. Management options could include which of the following?
i. Oesophagoscopy.
ii. Oesophageal swallow.
iii. Bronchoscopy.
iv. Left thoracotomy.
v. CT scan of the chest.
vi. Thoracoscopy.

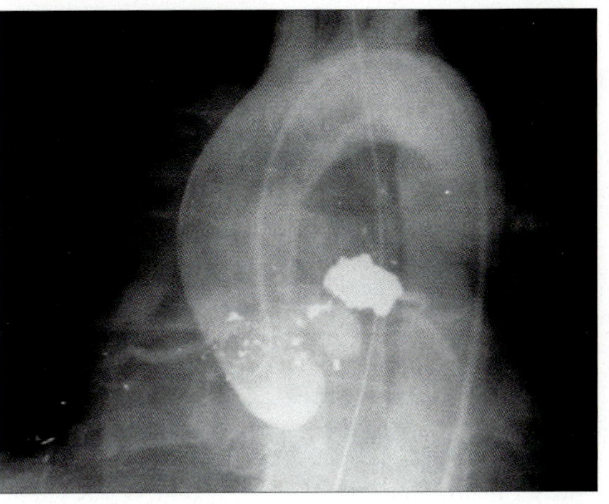

88 What two negative effects are common with all antidysrhythmics, which should be considered before administration?

89 A 26-year-old prostitute, known to abuse IV drugs, presents with *Staphylococcus aureus* pneumonia. A chest radiograph shows patchy bilateral pulmonary consolidation. She remains febrile despite 14 days of appropriate antibiotics. An echocardiogram is performed which shows large tricuspid vegetations. Discuss further management of this patient.

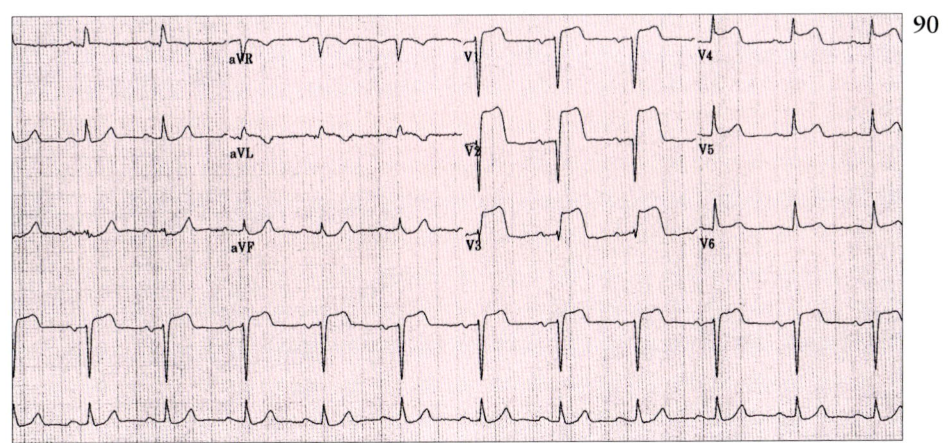

90 An ECG for a 62-year-old man.
i. What symptom might this patient complain of?
ii. Localize the abnormality.

87 Approximately 50% of patients with transmediastinal gun shot injuries are unstable on admission. Bilateral chest tubes should be placed and the side which appears to have the most blood draining be explored first. Median sternotomy is also an option, although exposure of posterior structures is difficult. Those patients who are stable require an extensive work-up. Aortography, oesophagoscopy and oesophageal swallow are required. Usually bronchoscopy is also performed but in a patient with no evidence of ongoing airleak or haemoptysis this is not absolutely vital. 10% of the original number will become unstable during this work-up, requiring urgent exploratory surgery, while about 20% overall will be found to have no thoracic injuries. A small percentage of these will have abdominal wounds requiring surgery.

88 All antidysrhythmic drugs have pro-arrhythmic side effects, as well as resulting in some degree of myocardial depression. The routine use of antidysrhythmics should be discouraged therefore, except when there are specific therapeutic goals.

89 Surgical intervention for tricuspid endocarditis is performed for severe embolic episodes, intractable CHF, persistent sepsis or myocardial abscess. Many of these infections are caused by virulent organisms such as *Staphylococcus aureus*, *Pseudomonas* and fungi, all of which are difficult to eradicate with antibiotics alone. Because of this patient's failure to respond to a reasonable medical regimen, surgery would be indicated. A point of controversy exists when the patient is also HIV positive, where definitive benefit of surgery is lacking. Several surgical options exist, including simple valvectomy, valve debridement and tricuspid valve replacement. Valvectomy is likely to be successful in the absence of pulmonary hypertension, although 20–30% will subsequently develop intractable right-sided failure. Debridement is not an alternative with annular or multileaflet involvement. Replacement risks prosthetic endocarditis, which is almost certainly fatal in these patients. Recidivism is high, and this influences the dismal long-term results in these often young people, with mortality rates of up to 90% at 5–10 years.

90 i. Chest pain.
ii. Dramatic ST elevation in leads V1–V4 suggest severe anterior ischaemia. The rhythm is normal.

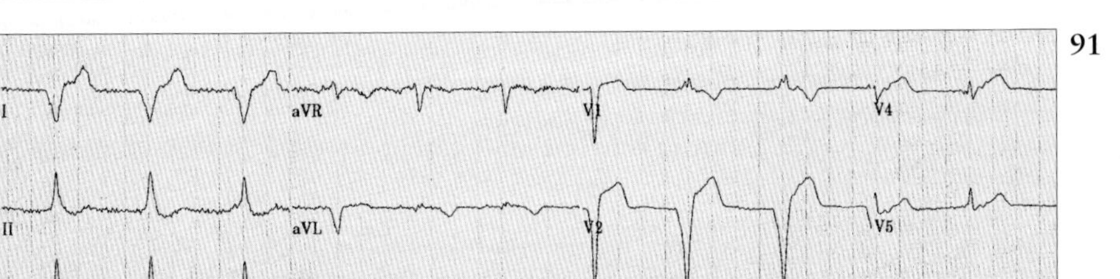

91 The same patient as in question 90 33 min later. His symptoms have resolved. What happened?

92 This patient had a chest tube placed because of subcutaneous emphysema and flail chest, accompanied by respiratory deterioration requiring intubation and ventilatory support. There is no air leak. What is the differential of the findings noted in this chest radiograph?

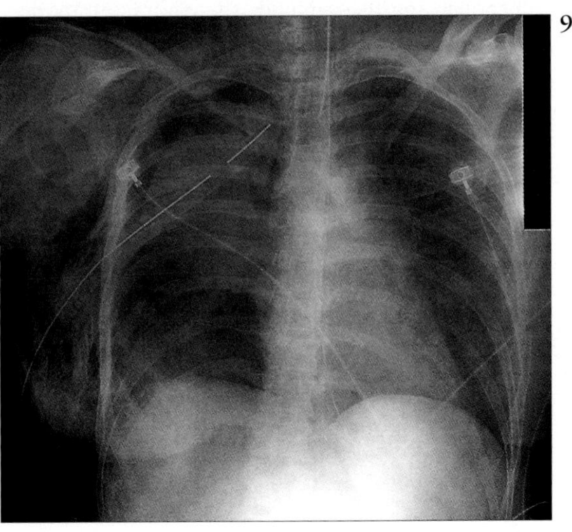

93 A 19-year-old man presents in cardiac arrest secondary to a severe asthma attack while playing basketball. The patient is quickly intubated and bilateral chest tubes are placed because of decreased breath sounds bilaterally. His downtime is 10 min since his collapse. Discuss the indications for left thoracotomy in this nontraumatic cardiac arrest patient.

91 Q-waves in leads V2 and V3 suggesting injury. There is also intermittent AV dissociation perhaps resulting from a competitive junctional or fascicular rhythm, probably originating in an injured or dying left anterior fascicle which gives a left posterior hemiblock pattern. Pain may be absent because he has completed the infarct.

92 The patient has a persistent pneumothorax without air leak. Mechanical causes include an obstructed tube (blood or kinking). Parenchymal causes include pulmonary contusion, pneumonia or other airspace disease preventing lung expansion. Bronchial causes include mucous plugging, intubation of the opposite mainstem or complete transection of the bronchus with mediastinal tissue obstructing the lumen of the bronchus.

93 Thoracotomy is well accepted for the penetrating trauma whose vital signs are lost during transport to the emergency department or whose vital signs are lost during resuscitation. Thoracotomy in blunt trauma is not well accepted. Indications for thoracotomy in medical arrests is controversial. Although the literature has demonstrated greatly improved haemodynamic profile during open cardiac chest massage over closed chest compressions, outcome has not improved in the human model. One reason is that open chest cardiac massage is not performed until closed chest compressions have failed which extends the downtime at least 20 min. Takino and Okada demonstrated that return of spontaneous circulation (ROSC) is time dependent and recommends that thoracotomy be done sooner (5 min after arrival to the emergency department) rather than later. ROSC rate was highest in patients with early thoracotomy and declined as the timing of thoracotomy was delayed. Further study is needed to determine if open chest cardiac massage, initiated concurrently with other ACLS treatment, has any role in the management of medical cardiac arrests in select groups of patients. Currently, it is not generally accepted.

94 Discuss the diagnosis and management of epiglottitis and LTB.

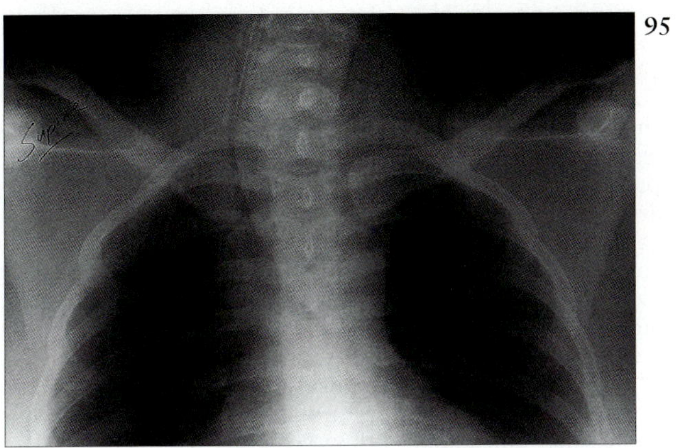

95

95 A 35-year-old man presented with a stab wound to the neck. His chest radiograph is shown (**95**). The initial step in the work-up and management of this patient is:
i. Angiography.
ii. Neck exploration in the OR.
iii. Observation.
iv. Local neck exploration in the emergency department.
v. Immediate intubation.

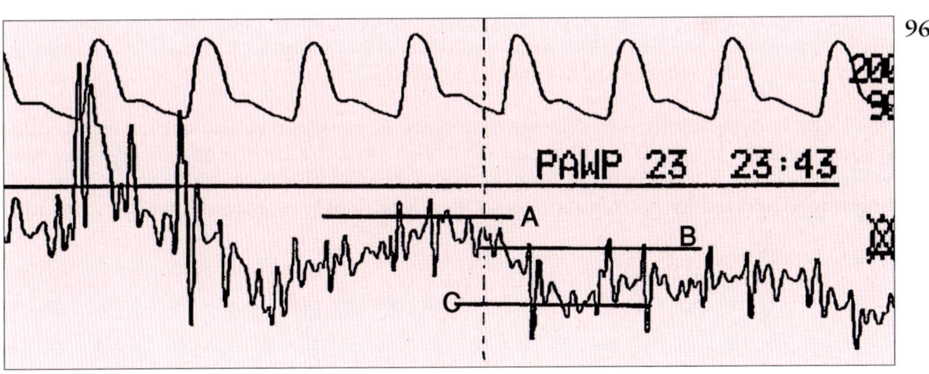

96

96 A tracing from a Swan–Ganz catheter during estimation of wedge pressure (**96**). The patient is intubated on pressure controlled ventilation mode and is not breathing spontaneously. Is the correct estimation of wedge pressure at point A, B or C?

94 Epiglottitis usually causes oedema of the epiglottis seen in the lateral neck projection as the 'dumbbell sign'. LTB is associated with the so-called 'steeple sign'. LTB may be confused with acute asthma. Epiglottitis is associated primarily with bacterial aetiology, primarily *Haemophilus influenzae*, while LTB is associated with a viral aetiology (parainfluenza in 75% of cases). Epiglottitis can affect all ages, but particularly in ages 2–7 years, and has a rapid onset. LTB affects those from 1 month to 7 years, primarily 12–24 months and generally has a more slowly progressive onset of 24–72 h after upper respiratory tract infection. Both present with dysphasia, stridor and chest wall retraction. Initial therapy is calming the patient down, supplemental oxygen and placing the patients in a sitting position. In any of these cases, whenever a patient is sent for any tests, a physician should accompany the patient to make sure there is adequate oxygen delivery and patency of the airway. The patient should be made NPO and IV fluids provided to prevent dehydration and insuppations. Racemic adrenaline should be considered as should systemic steroids. If epiglottitis is diagnosed, antibiotics that treat *H. influenzae* should be administered. Treatment might include the use of heliox. In settings of epiglottitis, laryngoscopy is generally considered to be contraindicated as it can cause spasm, although some centres with a great deal of experience are comfortable with fibre-optic examination. If intubation is required, it is best performed during deep inhalational anaesthesia without neuromuscular blockade.

95 v. Penetrating neck injuries present with moderately large or expanding haematomas requiring early intubation to prevent airway loss. The ideal intubation should be performed in a spontaneously ventilating patient with awake nasotracheal or oral tracheal intubation with or without fibre-optic guidance. If paralytic agents are required, only short-term agents such as succinylcholine should be used. Although one should be prepared to perform a surgical airway, this approach is associated with potential hazards of bleeding, injury to neck organs such as oesophagus due to distorted anatomy and contaminating a field where a vascular suture line may be required.

The angiography versus surgical exploration decision is made by the stability of the patient, the zone of the neck injury, and the clinical findings. Local exploration in the emergency department should be condemned.

96 C. By convention the PA occlusion pressure is measured at end expiration. In this patient who is intubated and ventilated with positive intrathoracic pressure the wedge pressure is influenced by ventilatory cycling. Position (A) reflects, in part, the pressure generated by the ventilator and therefore does not represent wedge pressure.

97 A 79-year-old man with bilateral rib fractures, pulmonary contusion, left haemo-thorax, and right acetabular fracture is in the SICU. He has the following haemodynamic parameters:

CVP 11 mmHg (1.5 kPa)
PCWP 13 mmHg (1.7 kPa)
CI 4.6 l/min
SVRI 1183
PVRI 223

Hgb 9.9 g/dl (0.99 g/ml)
Barometric pressure 760 mmHg (101.3 kPa)
FiO_2 55%

	Arterial blood gas	*Mixed venous gas*
PO_2	88 mmHg (11.7 kPa)	38 mmHg (5.1 kPa)
SAT	97%	69%
PCO_2	45 mmHg (5.9 kPa)	48 mmHg (6.4 kPa)
pH/[H$^+$]	7.44 (34)	7.43 (33)

i. The CvO_2 is: 20 volume %, 9 volume %, 15 volume % or 5 volume %?
ii. The $avDO_2$ is: 15, 10, 6 or 4?
iii. The alveolar arterial oxygen gradient is: 260, 410, 320 or 210?
iv. The shunt is: 15%, 24%, 31% or 5%?
v. The O_2 delivery is: 513, 483, 613 or 553?
vi. This patient's shunt is most probably secondary to: hydrostatic pulmonary oedema, aspiration, cardiogenic pulmonary oedema or pulmonary contusion?

98 A 47-year-old woman is admitted for an elective angioplasty of a proximal LAD/diagonal stenosis (**98**). After ballooning each lesion successively using a two-wire technique, the patient develops crushing chest pain. Discuss further management of this patient, with attention to indications for surgical intervention following acute angioplasty failure.

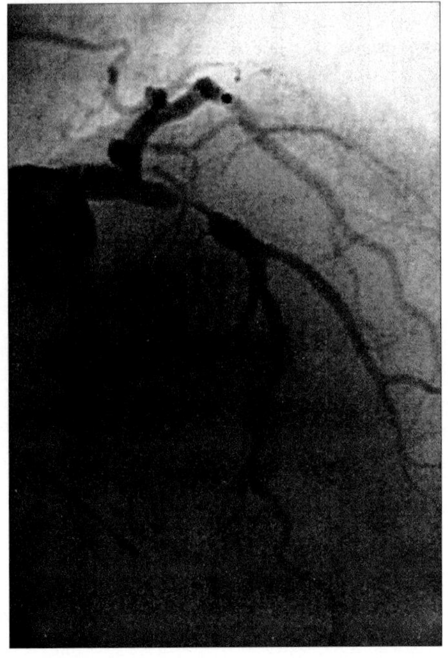

97 i. 9 volume %; **ii.** 4; **iii.** 260; **iv.** 24%; **v.** 613; **vi.** Pulmonary contusion.
The oxygen content of the arterial blood (CaO_2) or the oxygen content of the mixed venous blood (CvO_2) is calculated by the formula:

Oxygen content = Hgb × SAT × 1.37 + PO_2 × 0.0031

The oxygen content describes the amount of oxygen contained in 100 ml of blood (ml/dl or volume %).
Both oxygen which is attached to the haemoglobin and the oxygen dissolved in the blood are included. 1.37 ml of oxygen can combine with 1 g of haemoglobin. The $avDO_2$ or $C(a{-}v)O_2$ is the arterial venous oxygen content difference. This is a measure of the differences of oxygen content in the arterial and mixed venous blood. It is calculated using the formula:

$CaO_2 - CvO_2$

This difference is normally 4–5 volume %. The $avDO_2$ is elevated in low CO conditions such as cardiogenic shock, hypovolaemic shock or pulmonary embolus. High CO states such as septic shock or hyperdynamic circulation cause a decrease in the $avDO_2$.
The alveolar–arterial O_2 gradient ($aADO_2$) is the difference in O_2 tension in the alveolus and the arterial blood. The alveolar O_2 tension, depend on FiO_2 and barometric pressure.

A = FiO_2 (barometric pressure – 47 H_2O vapour pressure) – $PaCO_2$/0.8
$aADO_2$ = A – PaO_2

This gradient is normally 10 mmHg (1.3 kPa) in room air and about 70 mmHg (9.3 kPa) on FiO_2 of 1. An elevated $aADO_2$ is seen in pathological conditions associated with ventilation perfusion abnormalities.
The intrapulmonary shunt can be calculated by the formula:

$(CcO_2 - CaO_2) / (CcO_2 - CvO_2)$

or estimated from the $aADO_2$.
CcO_2 is the maximal CaO_2 at given FiO_2 and patient's haemoglobin. The calculated shunt is ca. 24%. To estimate the shunt from $aADO_2$ assumes that for every 70–100 mmHg (9.3–13.3 kPa) $aADO_2$, there is a 5% shunt. The patient's estimated shunt is 15%.
The O_2 delivery is calculated using the formula:

CaO_2 × CI × 10

There are four causes of pulmonary shunting in surgical patients: collapse, consolidation, contusion and water. The treatment of the patient with shunt depends upon the determination of the cause of the shunt through physical examination and chest radiograph.

98 Initial treatment usually involves further angioplastic interventions, with a view to reopening the vessel, or some method to provide temporary distal flow, such as a perfusion catheter. If cardiogenic shock is a feature, intra-aortic balloon pumping will be of benefit. The definitive treatment is expeditious transfer to the OR for emergency CABG, if the vessel cannot be reopened.

99 In the case **98**, the femoral artery was re-instrumented and angiograms showed acute occlusion of the LAD. Despite repeated attempts to cross the lesion, the patency could not be re-established and the patient continued to have ischaemia. Discuss the pertinent operative details in this patient.

100 A 30-year-old woman in her second trimester of pregnancy develops shortness of breath on exertion and is found to have mitral stenosis. Mitral valve area is 1.2 cm^2 on echocardiography. The optimal management would be:
i. Digoxin, diuretics and salt restriction.
ii. Warfarin (coumadin), digoxin and diuretics.
iii. Urgent closed mitral commissurotomy.
iv. Open mitral commissurotomy in the third trimester of pregnancy.

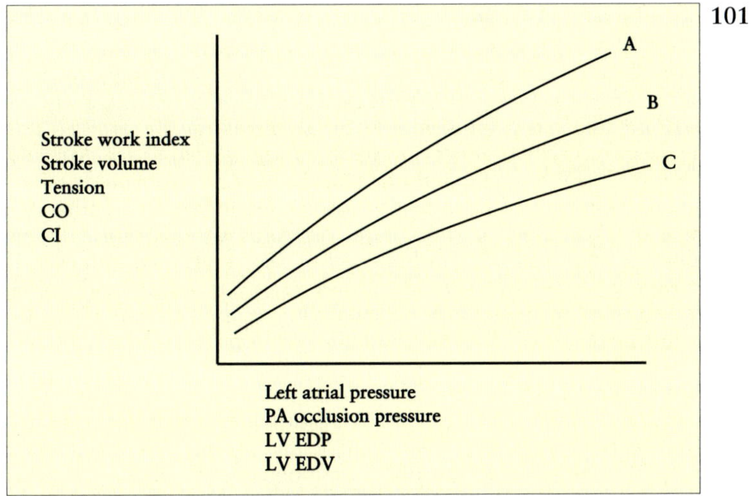

101 Three Frank–Starling curves are illustrated (**101**). If B is control, what could explain curves A and C?

99 The operative approach is based upon the degree of ischaemia, the haemodynamic stability, underlying ventricular function, comorbidity and the patient's age. Severe, prolonged ischaemia necessitates immediate institution of CPB, particularly if cardiogenic shock is present, in order to maintain adequate perfusion and to resuscitate the failing heart. Although the internal mammary may be taken down with the patient on pump, this is inadvisable in the very elderly, those with severe comorbidity, cardiogenic shock or severe pre-existing ventricular dysfunction, in whom vein grafts should be employed. Cardioplegia may be delivered antegrade successfully, but there is a theoretical benefit to retrograde delivery when coronary occlusions are present. Administration of various Krebs cycle substrates may be of benefit in resuscitating ischaemic myocardium. The primary consideration should be rapid revascularization of infarcting myocardium.

100 i. During pregnancy, labour and delivery the treatment of CHF is important, especially that of acute pulmonary oedema since this ranks as one of the most frequent causes of maternal cardiac mortality (accounting for 50% of deaths in pregnant women with rheumatic heart disease). At the early detection of pulmonary congestion, cardiac failure is best treated promptly and vigorously with marked restriction of physical activity, even bed rest, in addition to digitalis, diuretics and salt restriction. Aggravating or precipitating causes should be diligently sought and corrected. Coumadin has teratogenic potential and is ideally avoided during pregnancy. The need for cardiac surgery in this situation seldom arises. Mitral valvotomy without the use of CPB has a limited role and the only defensible indication is intractable pulmonary oedema and persistent massive haemoptyses in a patient with proven severe mitral stenosis. Open mitral commissurotomy would involve the use of CPB and introduces a major problem of high risk of fetal mortality, and even if the fetus survives it may be born deformed. There are scant reports of patients with mitral stenosis and intractable pulmonary oedema who respond to emergency open mitral valvotomy during the third trimester. Balloon valvatomy may be an option.

101 End diastolic fibre length can be estimated by end diastolic pressure, end diastolic volume or atrial pressure. The PAOC provides very indirect measurement of left atrial pressure, and hence of left ventricular pressure and volume, but is the commonest tool used to assess this on a continuous basis. Developed tension can be represented by stroke volume, stroke work or CO.

A shift to the right (C) implies that for a given fibre length, there is less tension developed. This implies cardiac dysfunction, as seen with ischaemia, heart failure or negative inotropes. One phenomenon described is 'diastolic creep'. This is the shifting of the curve to the right following temporary ischaemia, with gradual recovery of function and shift of the curve back towards control.

A shift to the left (A) implies increased inotropism, possibly due to the use of positive inotropes.

More direct measures include the use of left atrial pressure lines (usually post cardiac surgery), transoesophageal echo and/or right ventricular catheters (REVOX) designed to give volume data.

102 What is the difference between type A and type B lactic acidosis?

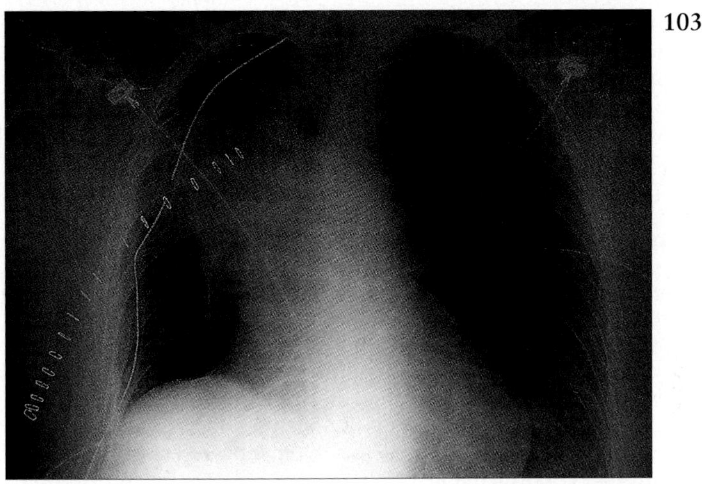

103

103 Following right upper lobectomy a patient becomes febrile and a chest radiograph shows consolidation of the right middle lobe (**103**). What are the diagnostic possibilities and what should be done to define the precise aetiology of the problem?

104 You have a young trauma patient in the SICU who is intubated and has a PAOC. Your clinical estimation of his haemodynamic status is that he is at point F on the Frank–Starling curve (**104**).

i. If all other parameters are kept constant and you give him a fluid bolus, at what point would you expect to be when it is complete?

ii. If this were an elderly vascular patient after repair of a ruptured aneurysm with known coronary disease and a history of congestive failure, what points could he be at?

iii. What sorts of interventions could change a person's haemodynamics to go from point F to point B?

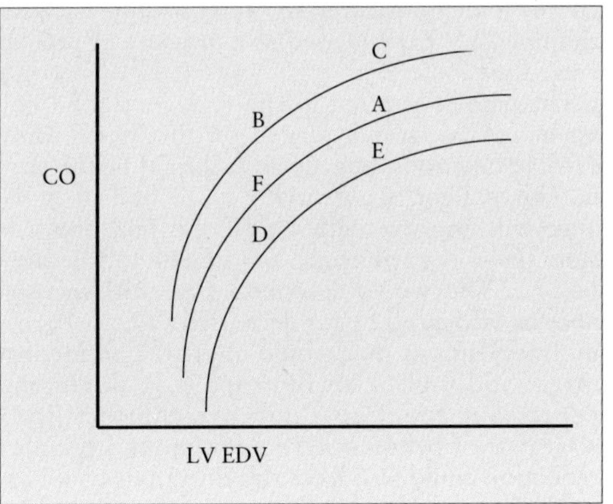

102 Type A lactic acidosis implies decreased oxygen supply due to poor tissue perfusion and/or hypoxaemia. It is the commonest form of lactic acidosis. Type B lactic acidosis occurs in settings when there is no evidence for decreased oxygen supply. Mechanisms usually involve increased production of lactate by glycolysis and decreased gluconeogenesis. Hydrogen and lactate production tend to be equal. Medical disorders include diabetes, renal and hepatic diseases, infections and leukaemia, related to drugs such as phenformin and occasional congenital forms.

Some information has been obtained experimentally by use of lactate/pyruvate ratios. Normal arterial lactate levels range from 0.5–1.6 mmol/l (0.5–1.6 mEq/l) and pyruvate levels 0.03–0.1 mmol/l (0.03–0.1 mEq/l). Increases in lactate/pyruvate ratio greater than 10:1 generally are taken to imply increases in the NADH/NAD ratio indicative of inhibited oxygen reactions which are consistent with tissue hypoxia.

103 A short period of aggressive pulmonary toilet should be tried to determine whether atelectasis is the source of the problem. If this fails to re-expand the lobe, a bronchoscopy should be considered. If the bronchial architecture appears normal after removing secretions, atelectasis is probably the source. However, if the affected orifice is fish-mouthed or the bronchial striations have a corkscrew pattern, torsion of the middle lobe should be suspected. Lobar torsion can occur spontaneously after trauma or pneumothorax, or in this case, after lung resection if the major fissure is complete. Lobar torsion usually pursues an inexorable septic course with the possibility of death unless an intervention is made. When the problem is recognized, thoracotomy is mandatory. If detorsion with return of viability can be performed, the affected lobe should be stapled to adjacent lung tissue for stability. However, in most instances the parenchyma will be gangrenous, requiring lobectomy.

104 This is the classic physiological relationship referred to as the Frank–Starling curve. It demonstrates the relationship between preload and contractility. In this example, LV EDV is used as a measure of preload with CO as one measure of ventricular function.

i. The patient at point F who receives a fluid bolus should have a rise in PCWP with an increased stretch placed on the myocardium of the LV resulting in improved cardiac function; thus, point A should be the correct answer.

ii. This patient is potentially more frail. If he is hypovolaemic his cardiac performance will improve with fluid bolus and point A will describe his new physiological state. If he is euvolaemic and unable to tolerate additional fluids he could end up at point E. This would describe a state with increased PCWP but poor cardiac performance as evidenced by his decreased CO.

iii. Interventions that would improve contractility without affecting preload are most often: addition of an inotrope (e.g. dobutamine, amrinone); removal of cardio-depressant could also improve contractility (e.g. emergence from anaesthesia, clearance of beta-blocker); addition of a peripheral vasodilator resulting in afterload reduction could also have this effect but could affect preload as well.

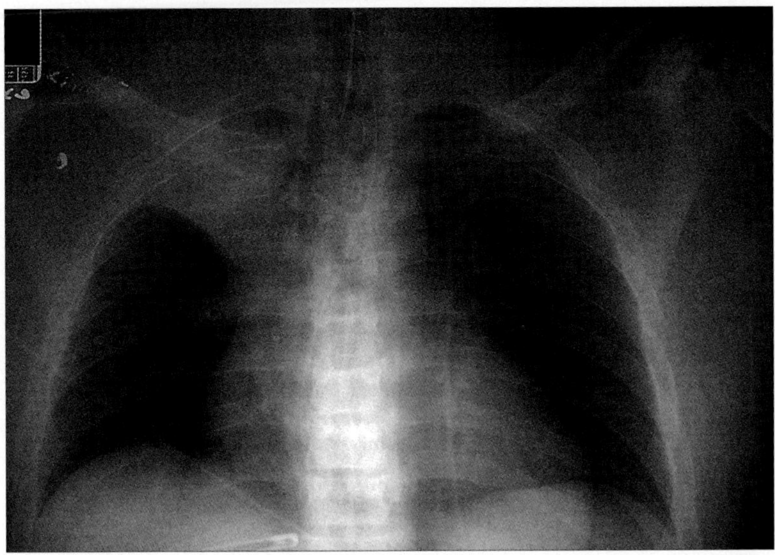

105

105 This 27-year-old man presented with a gun shot wound to the right supraclavicular area (105). There is a rapidly expanding haematoma necessitating intubation. The next best step in management is:
i. Angiography.
ii. Bilateral chest tube insertion.
iii. Supraclavicular exploration in the OR.
iv. Sternotomy in the OR.

106 What are the Class III antidysrhythmics?

107 A 72-year-old man presents to a peripheral hospital with an acute inferior MI, his chest pain having begun 36 h prior to admission. He was given streptokinase at a local hospital but continues to have ongoing severe pain, ST segment elevation, and evidence of pulmonary oedema. He is transferred to your institution where he is found to have a pansystolic apical murmur, evidence of cardiogenic shock and continued ST elevation, which prompts tPA administration. A PAOC is inserted and the following determinations are made:

	pO_2 mmHg (kPa)	pH (H^+)	FIO_2
Systemic	459 (61)	7.25 (55)	1.0
Pulmonary	78 (9.7)	7.17 (67)	1.0
Right atrial	56 (7.47)	7.18 (68)	1.0

Discuss indications for and outcome of surgery, as well as factors which influence survival.

105 iv. Penetrating injuries to the thoracic outlet are difficult to diagnose and manage. Ideally, arteriography should be performed as this leads to more accurate intra-operative management. Pitfalls in angiography include increased delay due to the time taken to prepare for it with the attendant risk of ongoing bleeding and arrest outside the OR. It should be possible to perform within 60 min. Angiography can miss arterial injuries and the associated venous injuries that occur in up to 33% of patients. Indications for angiography include penetrating injuries in the thoracic outlet, pulse deficit and neurological findings. Contraindications include instability of the patient, expanding haematoma and obvious arterial bleeding.

Some surgeons feel that all patients, particularly those with a haemothorax, should be explored through a supraclavicular approach rather than going to angiography. Patients with rapidly expanding haematomas, where the exact site of injury is not determined, are best approached by sternotomy which allows proximal control.

106 Class III agents include bretylium and amiodarone. These agents prolong all the phases of the action potential. Bretylium blocks noradrenaline release and can cause hypotension. It is used to treat refractory ventricular arrhythmias. Amiodorone has less pro-arrhythmic effects, has action against supraventricular dysrhythmias as well as ventricular ones, and has minimal direct cardiac depression. However, it has an extremely long half-life, and is associated with significant vasodilatation, which can persist for days to weeks. This can be particularly problematic following cardiac transplantation and may require maintenance with a vasoconstrictor for some days. Side effects include pulmonary fibrosis, hepatic dysfunction, bradycardia and occasional pro-arrhythmic effects.

107 The data reveal an O_2 step up beyond the right atrium. In this setting the diagnosis of post-infarct ventricular septal rupture is confirmed. Echocardiography can also make the diagnosis, but it can be difficult to obtain. Generally, the presence of such a lesion is an indication for surgery, particularly if severe end organ failure is not present. Without surgery, 25% will die in 24 h and 70% within two weeks. Delaying surgery in the hope of allowing the surrounding myocardium to become scarred and allowing more amenable suturing selects out those with the least haemodynamic alteration and deprives the larger proportion of patients a potentially life-saving operation. Preoperative interval correlates with increasing incidence of multiorgan dysfunction. Only those with small shunts (Qp:Qs<2:1) with very stable haemodynamics should be considered for delayed surgery. Inferior location, right ventricular infarction (common in inferior septal ruptures), elevated right atrial pressure, presence of cardiogenic shock, increasing age and early rupture following MI all have a negative influence on survival. Surgical results vary greatly depending on the reporting centre. Mortality for anterior defects is in the range of 20–50% and for inferior defects is approximately 30–80%, usually closer to the latter. Thrombolytic therapy is suspected of increasing the incidence of all forms of post-infarction myocardial rupture.

108 Discuss digoxin toxicity.

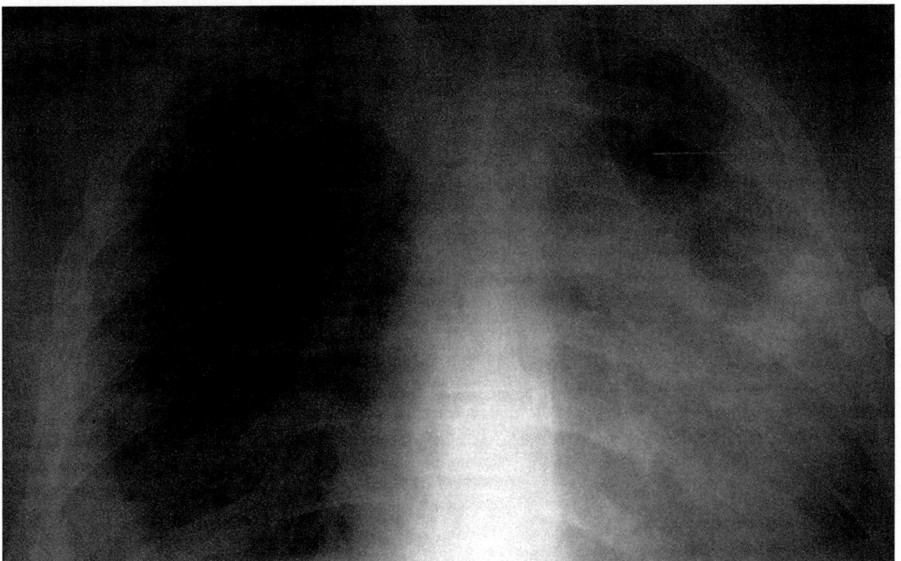

109 Following an emergency thoracotomy for a gunshot wound to the left lower lobe requiring a large wedge resection, post operative chest radiographs show a loculated air space in the left upper thorax (**109**). Chills and fever follow and a chest tube is placed documenting a staphylococcal empyema. How can this space be dealt with?

110 What is the cause of hypoxia in ARDS?
i. Interstitial oedema.
ii. Alveolar collapse.
iii. Shunt.
iv. Diffusion limitation.
v. V/Q mismatch.

111 Characteristics of congenital benign bronchoesophageal fistulas are:
i. Best treated by endoscopic techniques.
ii. Best treated by thoracotomy and division of the fistula.
iii. Usually present with symptoms in adulthood.
iv. Due to oesophageal inflammation.
v. Usually have a connection between the bronchus and the cervical oesophagus and are best treated by a cervical approach.

108 The risk of digoxin toxicity is increased in the following: the elderly; small body size; decreased renal function; hypokalaemia; COPD; in combination with quinidine. Clinical manifestations include loss of appetite and nausea. Serum digoxin levels are not useful in monitoring patients normally, because some patients require 'toxic' levels to control their heart rates and are not clinically toxic. They may be useful in initiating therapy if there are any of the aforementioned concerns. ECG changes include PVCs, atrial fibrillation with low ventricular response, Wenkebach phenomenon and/or RR interval becoming regular in the face of atrial fibrillation. Initial treatment includes withholding the digoxin, correcting risk factors, and administration of magnesium. In extreme cases, digoxin immune antibody (FAB) may be needed. This should be considered in the presence of life-threatening and progressive tachyarrhythmias, bradyarrhythmias resistant to atropine and serum digoxin level >10 mg/ml or potassium >5 mmol/l (>5 mEq/l). The dose is calculated by the following formula:

$$\{[\text{serum digoxin}] \times 5.6 \times ([\text{weight in kg}]/1000)\}/0.6 = \text{number of vials}$$

109 Drainage should be established with a chest tube. Thorascopic lysis of adhesion and drainage of the empyema is becoming increasingly popular as minimally invasive technology improves. If the patient is unsuitable for a significant operative procedure at that time, a rib resection with open drainage can be performed. Once the infection is under control, a decortication can be considered. If this is felt to be unreasonable due to dense adhesions, the cavity can be obliterated with transposition of a muscle flap such as the latissimus dorsi, pectoralis major, or rectus abdominis. Small space problems can be controlled with limited thoracoplasties.

110 This is a controversial subject. The complex nature of the pathophysiology and the controversies over primary pathological lesion of ARDS make this question difficult to answer definitively. The early pathology of ARDS is characterized by capillary leak, interstitial oedema and alveolar collapse. A component of shunt and VQ mismatch seems intuitive. There should be essentially three situations: normal perfused alveoli, nonperfused ventilated alveoli, and perfused but collapsed or diseased alveoli. Another controversial explanation of hypoxia in ARDS has to do with the platelet aggregation and micro thrombosis so inherent to the syndrome. As thrombosis progresses, cross-sectional area of pulmonary circulation decreases necessitating an increase in red cell velocity to maintain flow. As velocity increases diffusion limitation could be reached, i.e. the erythrocyte does not have enough time for complete gas exchange during a typical pass through the pulmonary capillaries.

111 iii. Congenital bronchoesophageal fistulas are due to a fistula between the bronchus and the middle one-third of the oesophagus. Almost all present in adulthood and should be treated by thoracotomy, division and interposition of a flap to prevent reformation of the fistula.

112 Fit the metabolic derangement with the ECG changes:
(a) Hypokalaemia.
(b) Hyperkalaemia.
(c) Hypocalcaemia.
(d) Hypercalcaemia.

(1) Prolonged QT due to prolonged ST segment.
(2) Flat T, increased QT and prominent 'U' wave.
(3) Peaked T waves (early state).
(4) Short QT due to short ST.

113 A patient requires a right pneumonectomy. History and physical examination reveal an unfit person in Class III NYHA status. The FEV_1, MVV, and DLCO are approximately 50% of predicted values. What further testing can stratify the risk of the proposed surgery?

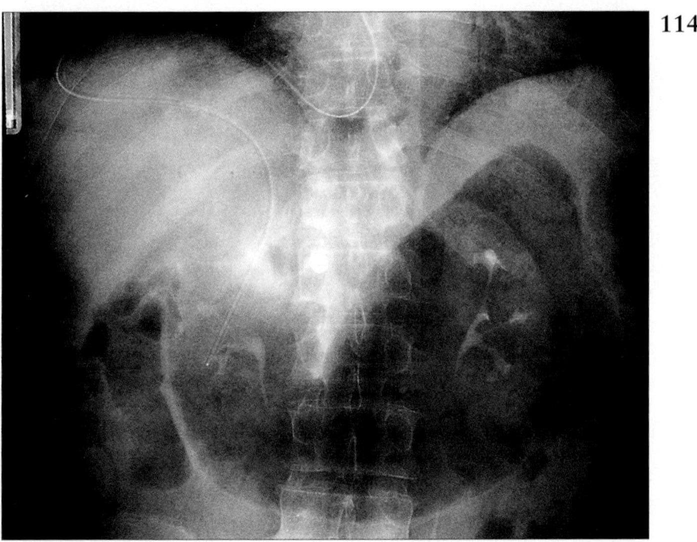

114

114 A 17-year-old man presents with a stab wound in the posterior left chest with stable vital signs. Chest radiograph after initial stabilization is shown (**114**). On the second day of admission, he developed fever, chills and chest pain. The next step in the management is:
i. IV antibiotics.
ii. Exploratory laparotomy.
iii. Left thoracotomy and drainage.
iv. Left thoracotomy and primary repair.
v. Cervical oesophagostomy.

112 (a) = (2); (b) = (3); (c) = (1); (d) = (4).

113 A patient requiring pneumonectomy should be able to climb two flights of stairs without extreme dyspnoea (should be able to count to ten without taking a breath) or undue tachycardia (heart rate less than 120 b.p.m.). A split perfusion lung scan should show a remaining FEV_1 greater than 800 ml or greater that 40% of predicted value. A patient with a maximal oxygen consumption (VO_{2max}) less than 10 ml/kg/min is unsuitable for significant pulmonary resection. Values between 10 and 15 indicate a moderate risk for postoperative cardiopulmonary problems. A value greater than 15 is rarely associated with significant perioperative cardiopulmonary morbidity or mortality. In patients with borderline values, a flow-directed PA catheter, capable of measuring RV ejection fraction, can be placed at the time of thoracotomy. Even if PA pressures are moderately elevated, a RV ejection fraction greater than 35%, a PVR less than 200 dyne/s/cm^5 or a PVR/RV ejection fraction ratio less than 5 should allow performance of a pneumonectomy.

114 **iii.** Traumatic oesophageal injuries are rare. The initial diagnosis may be suggested by mediastinal air, unusual placement of the NG tube as in this case, or confirmed by oesophagostomy or oesophagogram. These latter two are complementary tests as each miss 15% of injuries. Adjunctive ways of diagnosis including noting blood in the gastric tube or upon installing methylene blue noting drainage out of a chest tube. If untreated over 24 h, oesophageal perforation reaches a mortality of approximately 100% and primary repair will often be impossible. The best management is early diagnosis followed by a two layer closure and pleural or muscular flap reinforcement. This approach is recommended in the first 24 h after injury, but can be performed later if there is minimal pleural sepsis and the patient is stable.

A less satisfactory but reasonable option with delayed diagnosis is debridement, transpleural mediastinal drainage, and cervical oesophagostomy for diversion. Patients usually also undergo gastrostomy and jejunostomy. Currently, most thoracic surgeons advocate primary repair of the patient's overall condition is stable and there is no distal stricture. If there is associated stricture and repair is not feasible, complete oesophagostomy is recommended with interval reconstruction.

115 This patient suffered a stab wound to his heart with laceration of the distal LAD (115). Discuss methods of repairing penetrating coronary injuries.

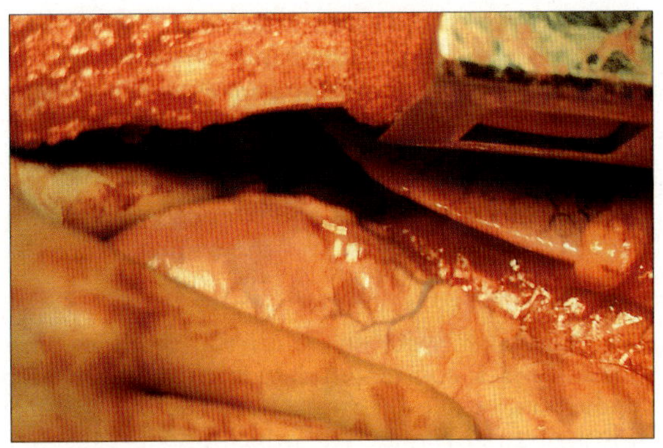

116 Discuss 'pacemaker syndrome'.

117 Which of the following are seen in the early microscopic pathology of ARDS?
i. Hyaline membranes.
ii. Complement deposition.
iii. Platelet microthrombosis.
iv. Interstitial oedema.
v. Inflammatory cell infiltration.

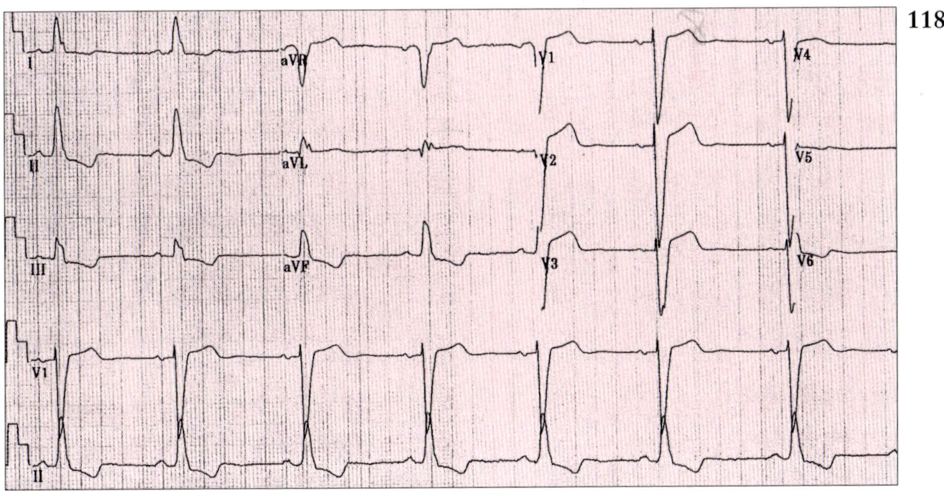

118 What is the conduction abnormality on this ECG (118)?

115 Coronary arteries are injured in 3–9% of penetrating trauma involving the heart, most commonly the LAD. Options include ligation if it is distal and small, primary repair or bypass using vein or internal mammary (off pump, on pump, and on pump with cardiac arrest). CPB and formal vein grafting appear to have a higher mortality rate (30–35%) but a lower morbidity (15%) compared to simple ligation. However, this is determined by the nature and site of injury. Most surgeons would ligate small distal injuries and consider bypass in the immediate perioperative phase after stabilization if there was evidence of extensive ischaemia and threatened myocardium.

116 Pacemaker syndrome is a term which encompasses a variety of symptoms, but generally is a consequence of ventricular pacing. Mechanisms can include VA conduction, setting up a re-entrant circuit or competing arrhythmias. These can lead to loss of atrial contraction (which provides up to 30% of CO and is critical in some patients), premature closure of the AV valves with resultant decreased CO and palpitations, or AV regurgitation. Other causes of tachyarrhythmias should be considered, including incorrect original diagnosis, metabolic and drug effects. The majority of cases have been attributed to retrograde conduction. In an extreme case, 'runaway pacemaker' resistant tachyarrhythmias and shock require disconnection of the pacemaker. The ventricular lead can be individually paced if required. In other cases, while correcting potassium and magnesium deficiency, ruling out other metabolic or pharmacological causes, the syndrome usually responds to reprogramming to eliminate the retrograde 'loop'. Reprogramming can also identify other problems, including inappropriate sensing, triggering, etc.

117 **iii, iv** and **v.** ARDS is characterized by lung oedema, microthrombi, inflammatory cell infiltration and late fibrosis. Hyaline membranes are characteristic of paediatric respiratory distress syndrome. Although complement deposition has been described in the pathophysiology of ARDS it would not be seen on microscopic examination.

118 Left bundle branch block. Note the delayed upstroke and wide QRS complex in leads I and V6. The atrium is in normal sinus rhythm with 1:1 AV conduction.

119 A 65-year-old man requires quadruple aortocoronary bypass grafting. He is noted to have a calcified ascending aorta. The best technique of revascularization should include:
i. Medical management only.
ii. Femoral artery cannulation and hypothermic circulatory arrest.
iii. Bilateral internal mammary implants (Vineberg procedure).
iv. Standard technique of bypass grafting.

120 Discuss the role of sodium bicarbonate administration in cardiac arrest or shock.

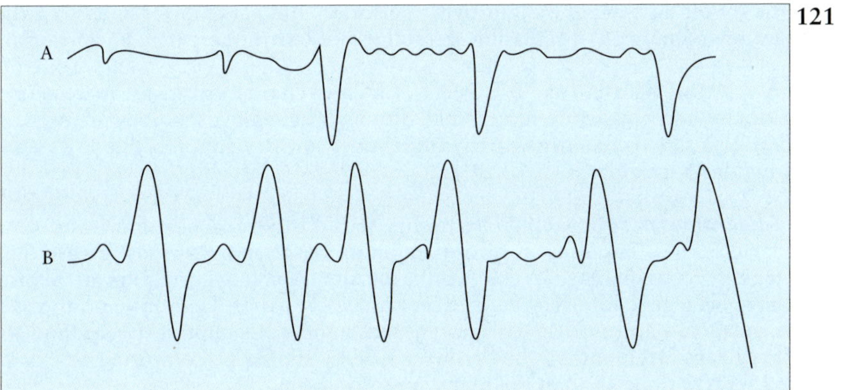

121

121 Which one of these ECG representations is atrial fibrillation and which one is MAT and why (**121**)?

122 A 73-year-old man presents with recent unstable angina and the cardiac catheterization demonstrates triple vessel disease. He had suffered an episode of amaurosis fugax 8 months prior to this. A cerebral angiogram was completed which demonstrated 80% stenosis bilaterally. Discuss the considerations in the surgical management of this patient.

119 ii. Calcification of the atherosclerotic ascending aorta represents a technical challenge to avoid a cerebrovascular accident. Intra-operative ultrasound is useful to identify location of plaque. To reduce operative risk for these patients, intra-operative Foley catheter has been used to occlude the aorta, modified aortic cross-clamp techniques, innominate artery utilization or Teflon for partial aortic replacement as site for proximal anastomosis, occasionally, ascending aortic atherectomy. Femoral artery cannulation and hypothermic circulatory arrest is a useful technique that obviates clamping and cannulation of the ascending aorta.

120 The treatment of acidosis with sodium bicarbonate is somewhat controversial. In patients with cardiac arrest with no real effective CO, it is thought that sodium bicarbonate may actually be harmful. This is because the pH [H^+] from ABGs are not reflective of venous and thus intracellular acidosis. Administration of bicarbonate may result in increased cellular acidosis and a worsening of cellular dysfunction. The acidosis should be treated by improving perfusion and ventilation. Following the restoration of spontaneous circulation, careful use of bicarbonate may be appropriate.

121 A = Atrial fibrillation. B = MAT. MAT is characterized by increased atrial automaticity and classically discernible, although changing, P waves are seen. Atrial fibrillation, a macro re-entrant arrhythmia, does not have appreciable P waves. Both are 'irregularly irregular'.

122 The surgical approach for patients with combined coronary and cerebral vascular disease is based upon prioritization as to the more serious disease (i.e. life-threatening) to be managed. The results for simultaneous correction of both problems have been generally very poor except in expert hands. Certainly in this case, due to the unstable nature of the coronary disease and the symptom-free period for the carotid disease (>6 months), the coronary surgery should be completed first, with the carotid surgery done at a later date if symptoms recur.

Several factors must be considered in the patient undergoing coronary surgery with significantly limited carotid blood flow:

- The mean perfusion pressure should be maintained relatively high (i.e. >70 mmHg (9.3 kPa)) during bypass.
- Systemic hypothermia should be considered due to its potential to decrease the extent of injury in the event of an embolic event.
- The management of the pH using the α-stat method has been shown to be associated with a lower incidence of neurological complications due to the relative cerebral vasoconstriction related to the decreased PCO_2 levels on bypass.
- Minimization of aortic manipulation and clamping.
- Subclavian artery stenosis may be present in these patients, thus precluding the use of the internal thoracic artery except as a free graft.

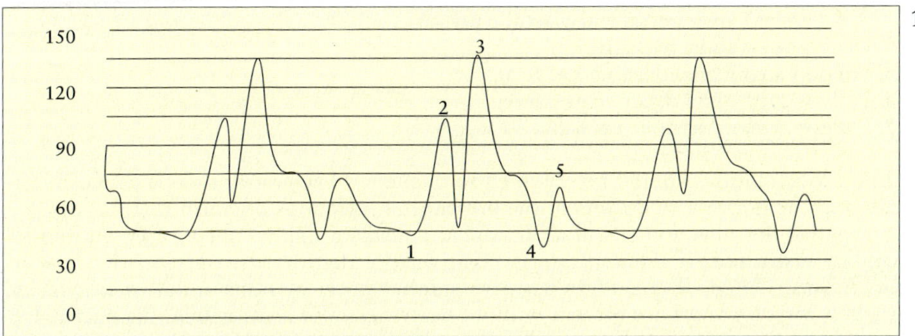

123 Representations of arterial tracings taken from patients with an IABP in place. What do the points 1–5 in (**123**) represent?

124 Several weeks following placement of a DDD pacemaker, the site of insertion becomes erythematous, oedematous, and tender. What kind of work-up and treatment should be instituted?

125 Six hours after being returned to the recovery room after an uneventful AVR, the following coagulation parameters were recorded in an elderly female patient:

INR   1.4
PTT   48 s
TT   44 s
ACT   185 s
Fibrinogen   1.4 g/l (140 mg/dl)

What process is causing these laboratory value abnormalities?

126 A patient with a severe hydrochloric acid injury of the upper GI tract:
i. Will require a gastrostomy alone if there is gastric necrosis.
ii. Has oesophageal sparing as acid burns only damage the stomach.
iii. Will require oesophagectomy alone with immediate or delayed reconstruction by the stomach.
iv. Has, as the main indication for laparotomy, abdominal tenderness.
v. Will require oesophagogastrectomy if gastric necrosis is found.

123 1. Patient's own aortic end diastolic pressure.
2. Unassisted systolic pressure.
3. Balloon augmented diastolic pressure.
4. Balloon aortic end diastolic pressure.
5. Balloon assisted systolic pressure.

124 Blood cultures should be obtained to document bacteraemia/septicaemia. Aspiration of the pocket can document the presence of infectious organisms. If the aspirate is negative but infection is still a prominent consideration, a course of IV antibiotics can be instituted. If the aspirate is positive, the therapy depends on the type of organism isolated. If coagulase-negative staphylococci or other indolent organisms such as *Streptococcus* are present without bacteraemia or septicaemia, the pacemaker pocket can be opened and debrided followed by a course of IV antibiotics. For more virulent organisms such as *Staphylococcus aureus* or Gram-negative bacilli, removal of all hardware is mandatory. If the lead resists removal, commercial extractors are available. These should be used only by experienced personnel since a risk of cardiac perforation with tamponade exists. In extreme cases an open procedure with CPB may be required to extract the lead system.

125 Extremely large doses of heparin are administered to patients undergoing open heart surgery. Much of this administered heparin will be bound by the endothelium and exposed subendothelium in the patient and will subsequently be slowly released back into the circulation. Thus, the half-life of heparin is proportional to the administered dose. After CPB, it has been estimated that heparin can be demonstrated in the circulation for up to 42 h after surgery. Heparin rebound results from the reappearance of heparin activity in the blood after the administration of an apparently adequate protamine dosage.

These laboratory abnormalities do not necessarily mean that the patient should be treated with protamine if there is no bleeding. In fact, it is likely that this low circulating level of heparin may be responsible for the extremely low incidence of deep venous thrombosis and pulmonary embolism in these patients. Further, overzealous correction of heparin effect in the blood may result in detrimental effects on graft patency. Finally, protamine itself, apart from the known potential haemodynamic and allergic side effects, may act as an anticoagulant in large doses and may inhibit platelet function, thus exacerbating bleeding. Therefore, this patient's treatment should be individualized depending on the extent of postoperative bleeding present.

126 v. A review of hydrochloric acid injuries shows that acid itself is more injurious to the stomach than the oesophagus. However, patients who require gastric resection often have associated oesophageal injury which causes either stenosis or further problems and are best treated by oesophagogastrectomy. Abdominal tenderness is a late sign of perforation and a much earlier indication of severe gastric necrosis is mental status changes.

127 Discuss the role of corrective surgery in a 6-month-old child with TOF.

128 A patient has a PAOC placed for haemodynamic monitoring. He developed right upper extremity swelling which prompted the study shown (128a).

A second patient has a central line placed for TPN (128b). He developed shortness of breath and fever.

A third patient develops frequent and refractory ventricular tachyarrhythmias (128c).

Describe the management of these cases.

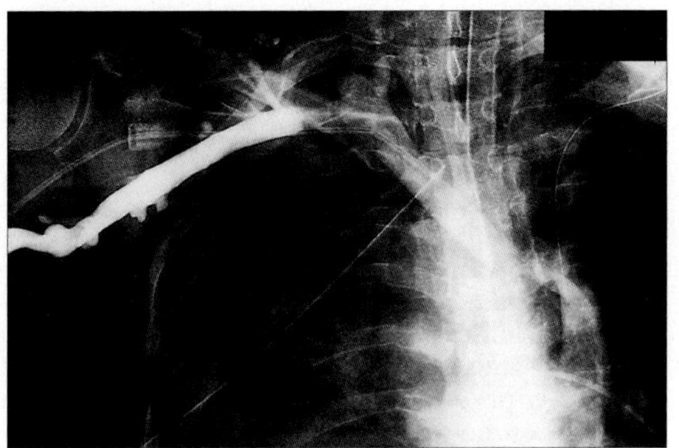

128a

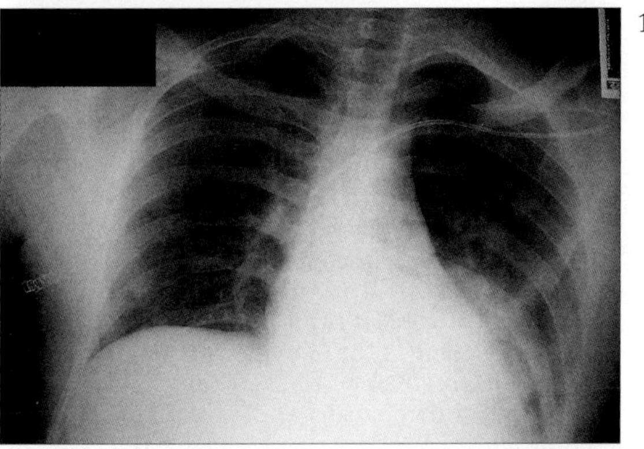

128b

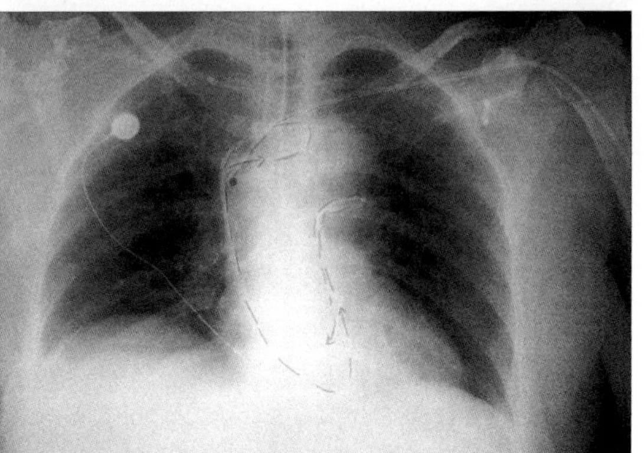

128c

127 Classic TOF includes an overriding aorta to the right due to a 'crystal' malalignment resulting in VSD and pulmonary outflow tract obstruction, both resulting in RVH.

Untreated, survival with TOF is 66% at 1 year, 49% at 3 years and 24% at 10 years. A subtype of TOF, associated with absent pulmonary valve with no atresia and unobstructed pulmonary flow, develops huge collaterals and death results in 50% by one year of age due to obstruction of bronchi by dilated pulmonary arteries.

Advantages of primary repair include: the avoidance of risk of palliative surgery and the subsequent risks of takedown; early relief of right ventricular strain; decreasing the complications of right to left shunt; and avoiding excessive left ventricular volume load. The initial palliative procedure, usually a B–T shunt, does have a lower mortality than primary corrective surgery however.

Most children who are >6 months of age are candidates for primary repair, while those less than 3 months, with medically refractory symptoms, are candidates for palliative shunts until they are big enough to undergo corrective surgery. Children between 3 and 6 months with medically intractable symptoms represent a grey zone. Patients with 'difficult' anatomy, such as pulmonary atresia, or small pulmonary arteries, or who may require a valved conduit, due either to pulmonary hypertension and or to a large coronary artery traversing the right ventricular outflow tract (5%), may do better with staged repair. Otherwise, primary repair is an accepted approach in these children at centres with a great deal of expertise.

With complete repair, there is <5% mortality, 1% heart block, and 5% need re-operation, usually for residual obstruction, VSD or conduit problems. 25 year survival is 95%.

128 The first patient (**128a**) has a subclavian vein thrombosis and a pneumothorax. Complications of central venous line placement include catheter malposition, dysrhythmias, air or catheter embolization, vascular injuries, cardiac injuries, pneumothorax, and brachial plexus injuries. The most common complication of any subclavian line placement is pneumothorax.

Second patient (**128b**): long-term complications include vessel thrombosis and line sepsis. The treatment of vessel thrombosis includes removal of the involved line, systemic heparinization and rarely thrombolytics. Complications with PAOCs include an increased risk of line sepsis, right bundle branch block (occasionally necessitating the need for external pacemakers in patients with pre-existing left bundle branch block) and knotting of the catheter in the right ventricle. Ventricular tachyarrythmias can occur, especially if there is malposition or wide loop of the PAOC (third patient, **128c**).

Another life-threatening complication is haemoptysis secondary to PA injury. The incidence is increased in elderly patients with pulmonary hypertension and in hypothermic patients.

129 What are indications for surgery in Ebstein's anomaly?

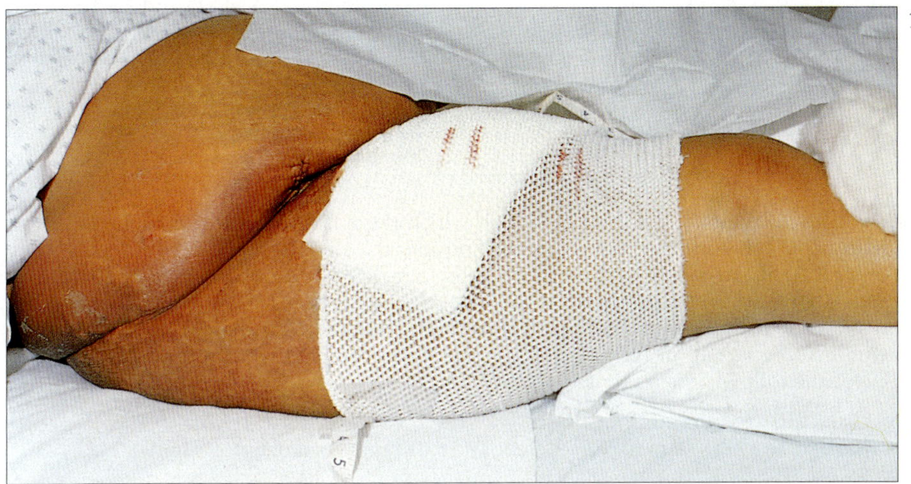

130

130 This 55-year-old man underwent elective cardiac catheterization through the femoral artery two days previously. He now presents with tachycardia, hypotension and thigh swelling as shown (**130**). The next step of the management includes:
i. Repeat angiography.
ii. Ultrasound.
iii. Operative exploration.
iv. Anticoagulation.
v. Fasciotomy.

131 A 20-year-old woman who had a coarctaction repaired 10 years previously, is shown on echocardiography to have a cleft anterior leaflet of her mitral valve with severe MR. The left ventricle is 56 mm maximal diameter in diastole. She is also shown to have a bicuspid aortic valve with a 20 mmHg (2.7 kPa) mean gradient and a residual gradient across her coarct repair of 15 mmHg (2.0 kPa). She denies palpitations, dyspnoea on exertion, orthopnoea or PND. Her mother claims she is very inactive. The results of an exercise nuclear ventriculogram show an EF of 56% at rest, rising to 68% with exercise (5.3 mets). Discuss the management of this patient.

129

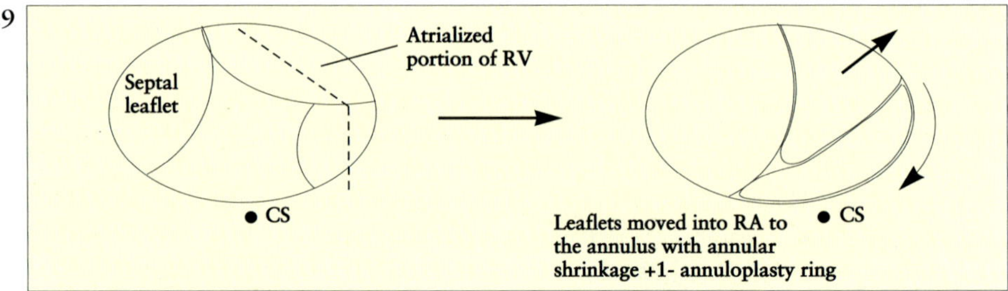

129 Ebstein's anomaly is a syndrome in which there is abnormal development of the tricuspid valve, such that the septal and posterior leaflets are displaced into the right ventricle. This atrialized portion of the right ventricle is thin and dilated and with the associated tricuspid regurgitation 'billows' during systole. This results in a loss of stroke volume and a degree of outflow tract obstruction. Most patients will eventually require surgery, but an increased death rate with medical management is described if one of the following is present:

- Class III/IV symptoms.
- Cardiac to chest ratio >0.65.
- Cyanosis or saturation <90%.
- Infant when diagnosis made.

Earlier surgery is usually recommended in this setting. Because of the 13% incidence of associated WPW (right ventricular free wall type), mapping is part of the evaluation. Surgical procedures described range from BT or rarely Glenn shunts for palliation of RVOTO to a procedure described by Danielson. This includes electrical mapping to allow concomitant correction of WPW, closing ASD/PFO, plicating the atrialized right ventricle, annuloplasty of the tricuspid valve or occasionally valve replacement. The Carpentier repair involves detachment of the anterior and posterior leaflets and relocation of the true annulus with or without concomitant annuloplasty.

130 iii. This patient has had a significant bleed into his thigh compartment that requires exploration. Operative approach should be through a groin incision. Proximal control may be gained by dividing the inguinal ligament or even a retroperitoneal approach to the external iliac artery. Primary repair usually is sufficient.

Complications of cardiac catheterization or angiography occur in up to 2% of patients and include bleeding, false aneurysm, arterial rupture, intimal dissection, embolization, and thrombosis of an atherosclerotic vessel.

131 Severe MR by itself is not an indication for surgical intervention. Although this patient has a dilated left ventricle, it is less than 65 mm and her systolic function shows a normal rise in ejection fraction with exercise. Reduction in exercise tolerance, CHF, ventricular dilation beyond 65 mm or loss of ventricular functional reserve are all indications for surgery. The onset of supraventricular arrhythmias is a relative surgical indication, but should be included in a patient as young as this, particularly if the valve appears repairable. In the presence of good ventricular function, an aortic valve gradient of 20 mmHg (2.6 kPa) is not significant. Likewise, a residual gradient of 15 mmHg (2.0 kPa) across the coarctation is about average and not of concern.

132 Discuss protamine reaction.

133 A 25-year-old man presented to a local emergency department following a stab wound to the right subcostal area. A radiograph is obtained (**133a**). A chest tube was placed (**133b**). There is no air leak. Why is the lung not expanding?

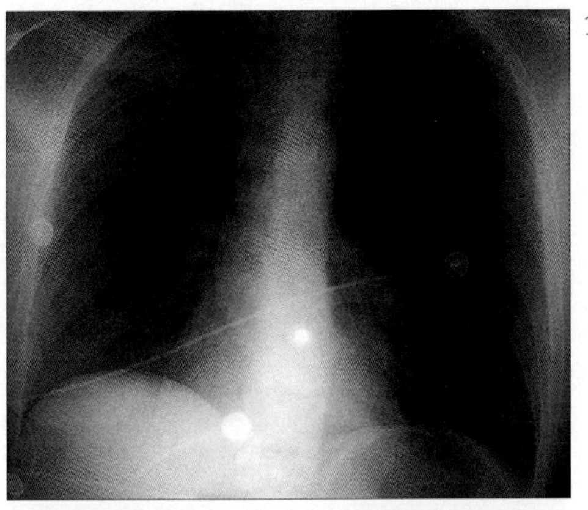

133a

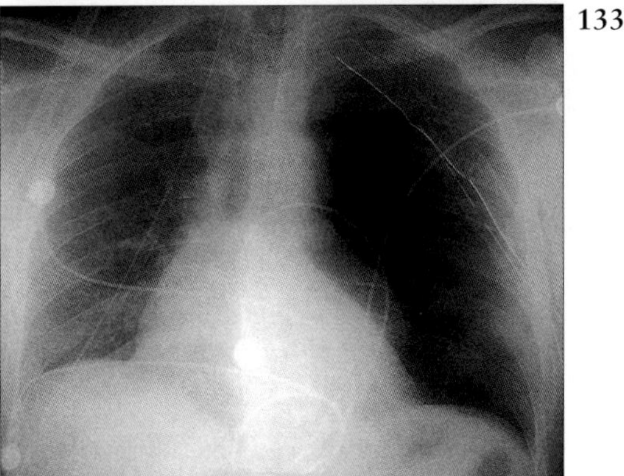

133b

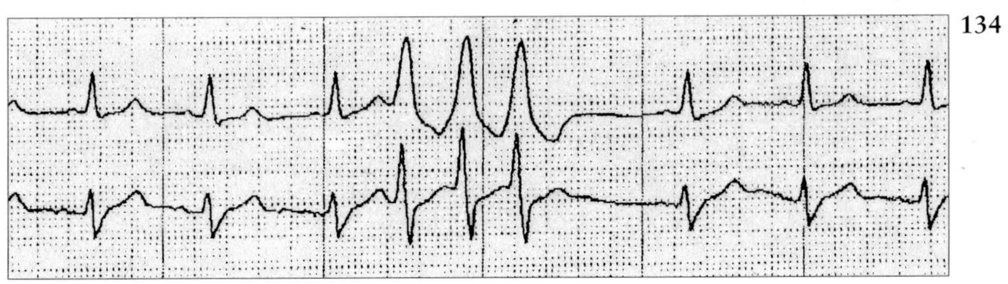

134

134 An ECG for an elderly man with chronic stable coronary artery disease awaiting inguinal herniorrhaphy. Describe the rhythm.

132 Four types of reaction have been described with the use of protamine that may cause hypotension:

* Dose-dependent non-allergic (this is uncommonly seen in patients receiving small doses of protamine; however, it can be prevented by slowing the administration rate of the medication).
* Dose-independent: anaphylactoid.
* Dose-independent: anaphylactic.
* Dose-independent: acute catastrophic pulmonary hypertensive crisis.

In the anaphylactoid and anaphylactic reactions, the patients become hypotensive related to the significant decrease in the SVR. The patient however will also have a significant drop in the right heart pressures (CVP, PA pressure) and there may be evidence of hives, oedema and bronchoconstriction.

Acute catastrophic pulmonary hypertensive crisis is characterized by a severe increase in the PA pressure associated with relatively normal left heart pressures. This is the situation represented in this clinical scenario and combined therapy with inotropic agents and pulmonary vasodilators such as PGE_1 and isoproteronol may be required. This is more often seen at the conclusion of cardiac cases.

Should open heart surgery be subsequently required in a patient such as this with a history of protamine reaction, several options are available:
i. In mild reactions, premedication of the patient 24 h prior to surgery with steroids, as well as H_1 and H_2 blockers appears to be effective in preventing this complication.
ii. If necessary, reversal of the heparin may be avoided after surgery; however, bleeding from the wound may persist and prevent sternal closure for some time.
iii. Several alternatives to heparin may be used during surgery such as prostacyclin analogues.
iv. Heparin-removal devices involving immobilized heparinase are effective and are now available.
v. Platelet factor IV rapidly binds heparin in circulation. This product is available in a recombinant form and has recently been shown to be effective in completely reversing heparin levels after CPB.

133 This patient has a large bulla. The first radiograph demonstrates lung markings in the lower half of the lung field, with a curved aspect as if it were being compressed. Failure of a pneumothorax to resolve can be attributed to a plugged or misplaced tube, bronchial obstruction or disruption, or to the fact that there never was a pneumothorax. Parenchymal disease (e.g. contused lung/prolonged collapse) may also prevent re-expansion. The differential of hyperlucent spaces includes congenital defects (e.g. lobar emphysema, adenomatous malformation, absence of lung tissue) and acquired (air cysts from obstruction, blebs and bullae etc).

134 A triplet of three PVCs during otherwise normal sinus rhythm. Note that the QRS complex is wide. Although P waves are clearly recorded preceding normal QRS complexes, there are no P waves preceding the PVCs. There is a compensatory pause after the last PVC.

135 List ECG characteristics of aberrant ventricular conduction and ventricular ectopy.

136 Discuss the evaluation and management of patients with thymic tumour (**136**).

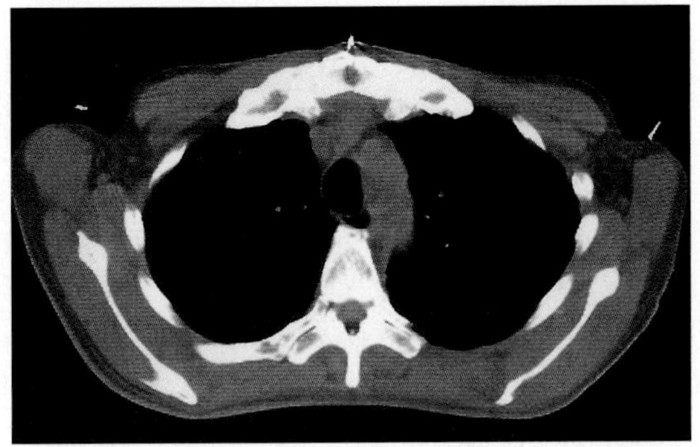

136

137 What is the abnormality in this ICU chest radiograph (**137**)?

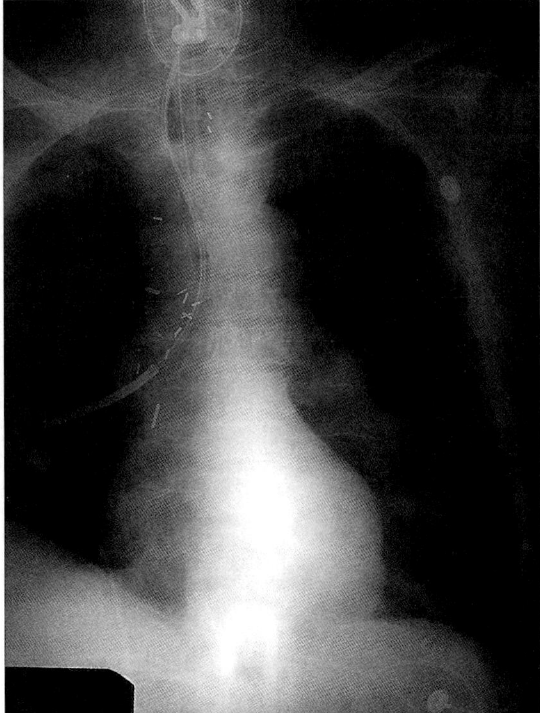

137

135 Aberrant ventricular conduction is associated with the following: RBBB with R' > R in V1; R rate = 170/min; intrinsic QRS vector = conducted QRS vector; QRS <140. ventricular ectopy is associated with the following: LAD; QRS >140; mono or biphasic V1; fusion or capture beats; rate <170 b.p.m.; AV dissociation; R>R' in V1.

136 Regular chest radiographs and CT of the chest (**136**) can show the relationship of the anterior mediastinal mass to contiguous structures. A work-up should be performed to detect the presence of myasthenia gravis. If this autoimmune disease is documented, consider the use of anticholinesterase medications such as pyridostigmine. Corticosteroids, plasmapheresis, and immunosuppression are usually reserved for recalcitrant or nonoperative cases. Medications that should be avoided during the perioperative period include anticholinesterase inhibitors in large doses (cholinergic crisis), chlorpromazine, clindamycin, gentamycin, lidocaine (lignocaine), phenytoin, procainamide, propranolol, thyroid hormones and trimetaphan. In the operating room, avoid depolarizing muscle relaxants such as succinylcholine. If muscle relaxation is required use short-acting, nondepolarizing agents such as atracurium or vecuronium. Avoid inhalation agents such as isoflurane, methoxyflurane or enflurane. The following may indicate the need for prolonged mechanical ventilation following thymectomy for myasthenia gravis: duration of myasthenia greater than 6 years; coexistent pulmonary disease; pyridostigmine dose greater than 750 mg/day or an FVC less than 2.9 l. In general all thymic tissue should be removed when possible. Cervical thymectomy often leaves residual thymic tissue. Median sternotomy seems to offer the best approved to the anterior mediastinum. The role of thymectomy via thorascopy is currently under investigation.

137 This patient has a feeding tube which has been placed in the trachea. It now rests a main stem bronchus. All feeding should be stopped and it should be removed immediately. This is a more common problem when placing narrow gauge nasoenteral feeding tubes because they are less stiff then the traditional Levin NG tube and are often placed in intubated patients with alterations in mental status. Methods to avoid this problem include: use a tube with a wire guide during placement for greater stiffness; do not force the placement; try different positions of head and neck if the tube does not pass easily; always check placement before feeding (this can be done by instilling air while auscultating with a stethoscope or some people would use radiographic confirmation for all feeding tubes); since the ideal placement for feeding is beyond the pylorus some would argue that placement should occur in the radiology or endoscopy suite to avoid morbidity and eventually decrease cost.

138 A 35-year-old man presents with massive haematemesis. Ten years previously he had suffered a gunshot to the upper abdomen that required debridement of the left lobe of the liver, and 'trauma Whipple', including antrectomy and Bilroth II. On a previous admission, also for upper GI bleed, gastric pH was documented as being 1.0 ($[H^+]$ >75), and he was started on H_2 blockers but was non-compliant. An EGD reveals an ulcer close to the anastomosis (138). He rebleeds despite intense medical management and then stabilises. It is felt that he may have had an incomplete vagotomy. Discuss the 'best' approach for this.

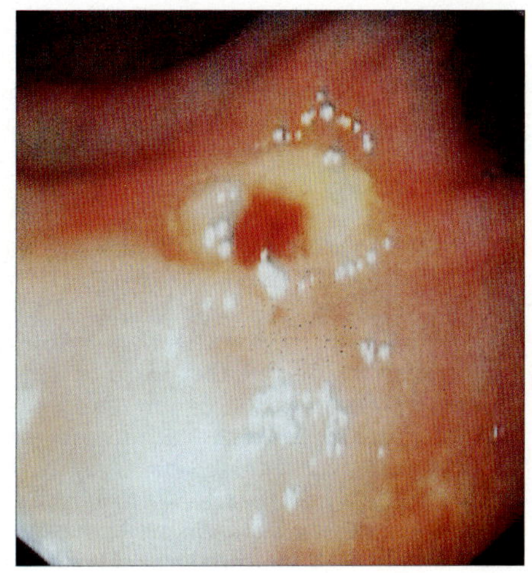

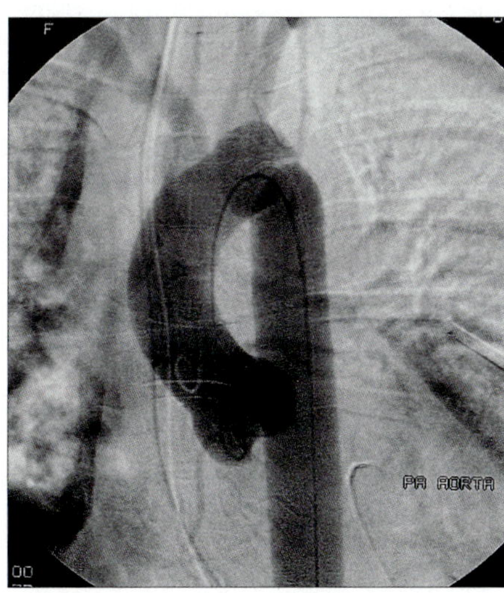
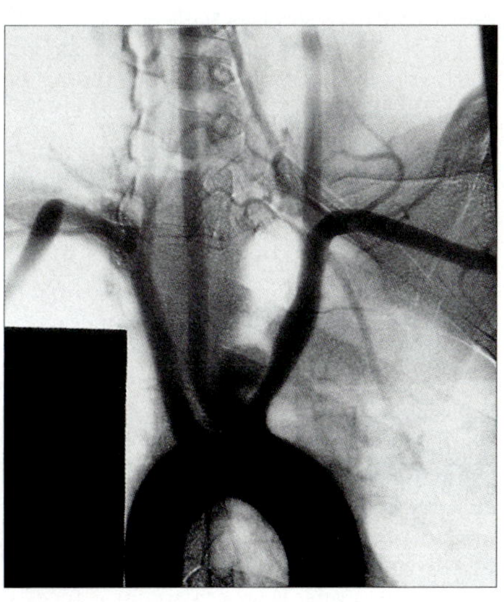

139 Discuss the medical and surgical management of the patients whose arteriograms were obtained following RTAs (139a, b).

140 A 66-year-old man presents with unstable angina eight weeks following reoperative CABG where a LIMA was placed to the LAD and a vein graft to the distal RCA. Repeat angiography shows a tight stenosis of the proximal aorto-saphenous anastomosis. Discuss the therapeutic options for this patient.

138 It was felt that this patient needed surgery because he had rebled three times, the last on medical management. Because of the extensive upper abdominal surgery, it was elected to perform the vagotomy through a left thorascopic approach. Other options include a repeat abdominal approach, possibly with further gastric resection to ensure that there is no retained antrum. In a patient with his surgical history, this would be a formidable undertaking.

139 Traumatic deceleration injuries to the thoracic aorta cause death at the scene in 85% of patients. Of the 15% who survive to come to a trauma centre, 40% will die within 24 h. Once recognized, initial treatment includes controlling heart rate and blood pressure. In an otherwise stable patient, with no other injuries requiring surgery, Labetolol, or other short acting beta-blockers are ideal. Some patients may not be operative candidates initially. Reasons include: lung injuries that preclude one lung ventilation; severe myocardial dysfunction; severe CNS injuries that preclude ultimate survival. Ideally, these patients are managed in an ICU, possibly with transthoracic echo monitoring of both cardiac function and the haematoma. The majority of patients should be operated on with relative emergency. Arterial pressures should be monitored via the right radial artery. The approach requires a left posterolateral fourth interspace thoracotomy with independent lung ventilation. Control of the left subclavian artery and aorta between the left subclavian and common carotid vessels as well as and distal to the haematoma is obtained. Controlling the aorta proximal to the left subclavian is important because in a number of cases the tear will extend proximal to the origin of the left subclavian (as shown in **139b**).

Paraplegia occurs postoperatively in up to 15% of patients. The most critical determinant is the duration of the cross clamp time, which should be ideally less than 45 min. The use of heparin-bonded pumps (Biomedicus) can be useful.

140 Early recurrence of angina following CABG is uncommon, but does occur in about 2% of cases, and is usually the result of technically inadequate graft construction, although accelerated fibrointimal hyperplasia may rarely be the cause. Therapeutic options for this patient include anti-anginal medication, percutaneous graft interventions and repeat surgery. If angina is easily controlled with medication, this would probably be an accepted course of action. Unfortunately, this is usually not the case. Catheter interventions include angioplasty, stenting and rotablation, frequently in combination. Balloon angioplasty is difficult at the aortic take-off of saphenous vein grafts and has a very high rate of early restenosis (approaching 70% at 6 months). Stenting appears to reduce restenoses after balloon angioplasty, but is not an option in this case as the stent would be precariously placed across the ostium of the vein graft. Rotablation is probably in this instance the most durable of the catheter options. Reoperation at 6 weeks would be exceptionally difficult because the vascularity of the adhesions and the friability of the tissues, and would thus be a last resort.

141 Discuss peri-operative management of a patient with HLHS who is to undergo a Norwood procedure.

142 Describe surgical techniques possible in repairing penetrating cardiac injuries.

143 A 2.6 kg male infant is transferred following an uneventful pregnancy and delivery. A diagnosis of oesophageal atresia and tracheoesophageal fistula is made by failure of a nasal tube to reach the stomach (**143**). Other anomalies that may be associated with this condition include:
i. Vertebral anomalies.
ii. Imperforate anus/anorectal agenesis.
iii. Deformities of the radial ray of one or both upper limbs.
iv. TOF.
v. All of the above.

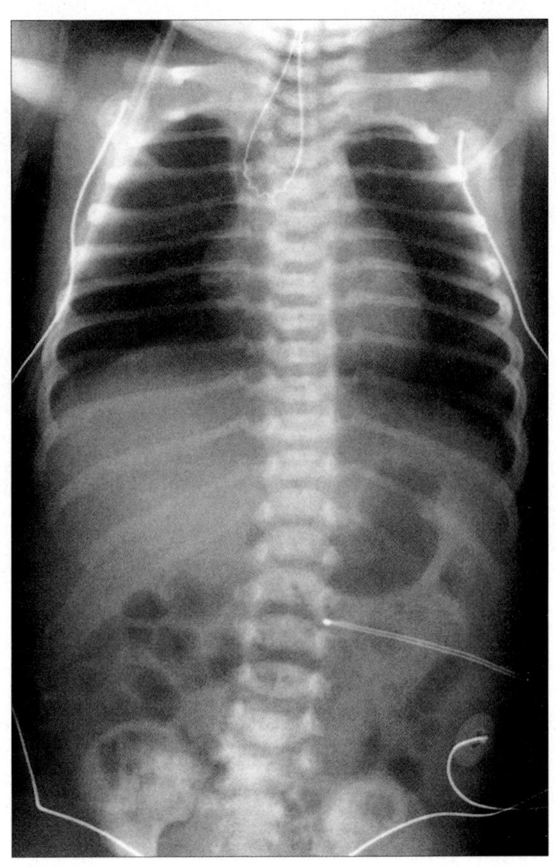

141

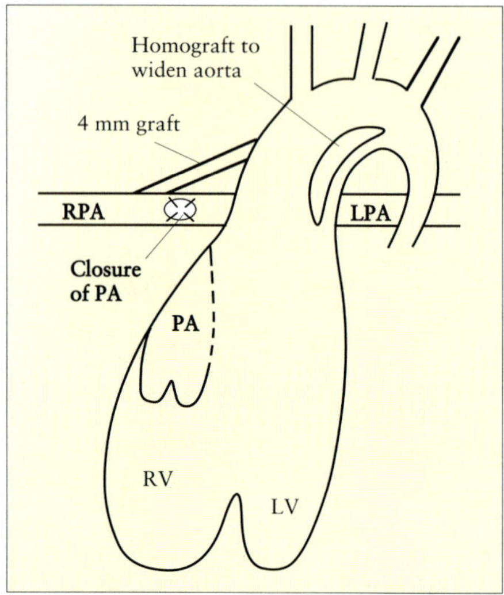

141 HLHS is a syndrome characterized by aortic atresia or stenosis, mitral stenosis (60%) or atresia (40%) and a diminutive left ventricle. Systemic flow is maintained by perfusion retrograde through the PDA. Rarely, there is a nonrestrictive VSD such that the LV is relatively normal. Dr Norwood described a two-stage procedure, as an alternative to compassionate care only or heart transplantation. The first procedure involves creating a neo-aorta out of the PA, with additional homograft, and using a shunt to connect the PA to this new systemic outflow. This shunt is usually a 4 mm Goretex graft which limits pulmonary flow (**141**). When PVR drops sufficiently (usually 18 months) a Fontan is performed. Overall survival may be as low as 25% or less however.

Prior to the initial phase, the patency of the ductus is maintained with PGE_1. It is important to maintain PVR at an elevated level, as dropping it will steal from systemic flow, thus $PaCO_2$ is maintained at 45–50 mmHg (6.0–6.7 kPa). Septostomy should not be performed as long as the PaO_2 is greater than 25 mmHg (3.3 kPa), as this will reduce the pulmonary venous resistance, which will in turn reduce PVR. Following surgery, the goal is to maintain systemic saturations of 75–80%, which represents balanced pulmonary and systemic flow.

142 Of penetrating cardiac injuries, the right ventricle is reported to be affected in 35% of cases, the left ventricle in 25%. Initial control can be obtained by using digital pressure, a 30 ml Foley catheter (avoiding excessive traction that could extend the tear) or skin staples. The atria can be clamped with vascular instruments but clamps should be avoided on the ventricles. Following initial control, injuries to the ventricles can be primarily repaired using pledgeted (pericardial or Teflon) 3-0 Ethibond, silk or proline. The atria can often be repaired with a figure of eight or running suture.

CPB may play a role in an acidotic, hypothermic patient who, having undergone urgent thoracotomy with control of the injury, needs to be rewarmed and have acidosis reversed.

143 v. The VATER syndrome is the nonrandom association of various anomalies first described by Quan and Smith in the 1970s. Vertebral anomalies, anorectal anomalies, tracheoesophageal anomalies, and abnormalities of the radial ray of one or both upper limbs are all commonly associated. In addition, cardiac and renal abnormalities are also seen. The primary importance of this association is the possibility of other abnormalities when presented with a child with one of these anomalies.

144 Discuss the differential diagnosis of a posterior mediastinal mass in a hypertensive patient.

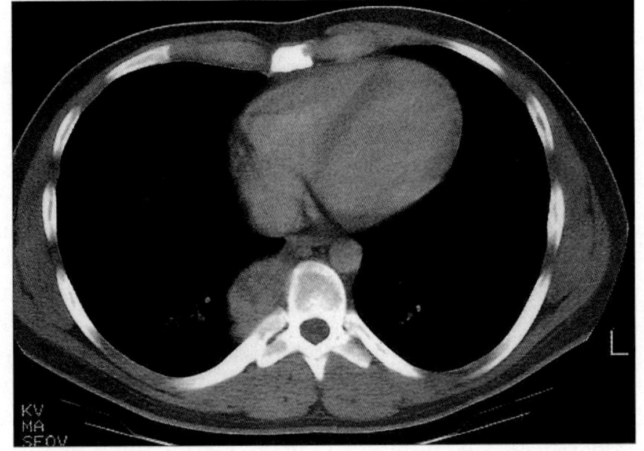

145 What are the options available to a patient with a recurrent spontaneous pneumothorax?

146 What is the abnormality in this ICU chest radiograph (**146**)?

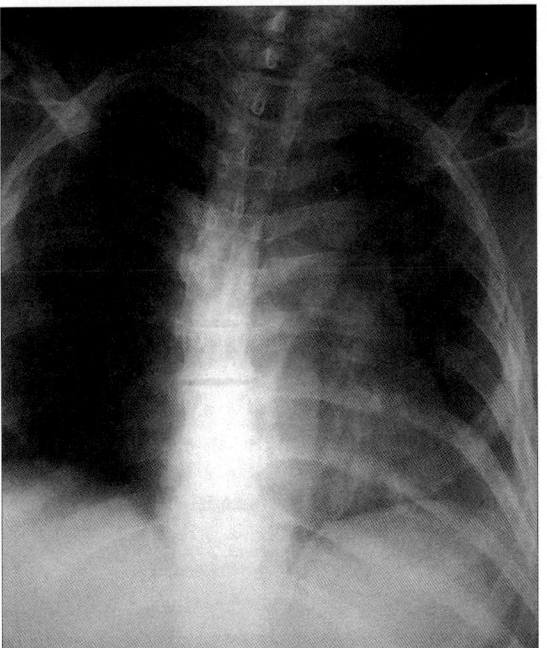

144 The most common posterior mediastinal masses include oesophageal duplication cysts and neurogenic tumours. However other aetiologies such as mediastinal pheo-chromocytoma (paraganglioma) should be considered in those with hypertension associated with diabetes mellitus or a hyperdynamic state. Urine vanillylmandelic acid >10 mg/24 h is diagnostic of this problem. In patients with hormonally active tumours, alpha-adrenergic blockade with phenoxybenzamine should be instituted for 2 weeks. Also, consider beta-adrenergic blockade with propranolol. Indicators of good blockade include control of hypertension, presence of postural hypotension, resting tachycardia, and thirst. In the operative setting avoid atropine, morphine, curare, atracurium, pancuronium, succinylcholine, ephedrine, chlorpromazine, and metoclopramide. In the OR have short acting vasodilators such as nitroprusside and beta-adrenergic agonists available. For treatment of hypotension after resection, vasopressors should be immediately available.

145 Since the likelihood of repeated pneumothorax is increased with the second occurrence, observation alone is a poor choice. However if this is elected, the use of supplemental oxygen by mask or nasal cannula may speed its re-absorption. Simple aspiration can control the pneumothorax, but recurrence is likely. A CASP/chest tube should be inserted in symptomatic patients or with larger pneumothoraces (greater than 20%). Sclerotic agents such as doxycycline or talc can be used, but the long-term effectiveness and side effects are still not known. Thoracoscopy or definitive muscle sparing thoracotomy with pleurectomy and bulla stapling/ligation would seem to offer the best chance of controlling recurrent pneumothorax.

146 The differential diagnosis of the abnormalities is film is large. However, the trite abnormality is poor radiological technique. The patient is rotated on this film and the subsequent chest radiograph was found to be normal. It all too easy to forget the basics of reading films in the ICU in the rush to complete an endless list of tasks; the radiographs are viewed with specific abnormalities in mind and subtle changes are missed. A systematic approach to reading films is imperative. It should always begin with verification that the correct patient has been filmed and a comment on the technique and quality of film (post, penetration, etc). Subsequent analysis is based on personal preference, a useful mnemonic is A-B-C: Abdomen (bowel gas pattern, position of NG or feeding tube, free air, etc.), Bones (missed rib, clavicle, or scapular fracture in trauma patients), Chest (heart, lungs, tubes and lines, etc). Comparison with previous films, when available, is always useful.

147 A 56-year-old woman presented after a RTA with evidence of a widened mediastinum (147). Arteriography revealed the lesion shown. She is asymptomatic. Discuss the management of this patient.

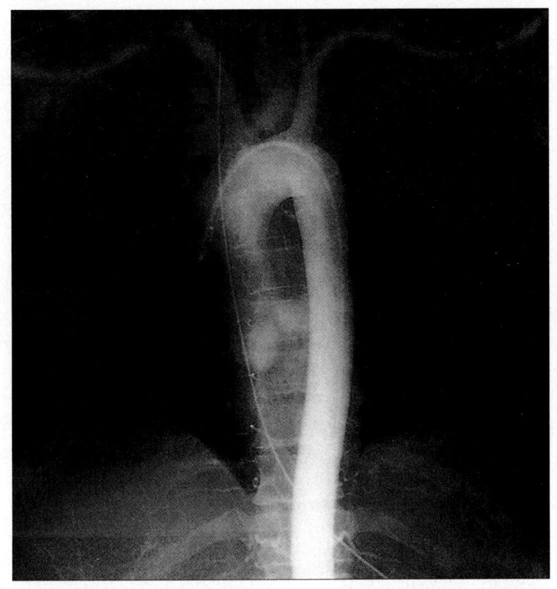

147

148 Aortic incompetence associated with acute type A dissection could be managed by which of the following:
i. Modified Bentall operation only.
ii. Repair of aortic dissection and aortic valve repair where possible.
iii. Repair of ascending aortic dissection and IABP support.
iv. Medical treatment using afterload reduction.

149 A 30-year-old female is admitted to the ICU following a RTA. An exploratory laparotomy showed a splenic laceration which was suture repaired and a small pelvic haematoma. She also underwent internal fixation of her left femoral fracture. Her pelvic radiograph revealed a left superior and inferior ramus fracture. She had on chest radiograph a left pulmonary contusion with rib fractures 4, 5 and 6. She is being ventilated on 60% FiO₂, a PEEP of 10 cm H₂O, a rate of 12 breaths/min, and a tidal volume of 800 ml. She was reported to be stable during the surgical procedure. Her ventilatory pressure suddenly increases, the high pressure alarm goes off and the patient begins desaturating. The most likely aetiology is:
i. Worsening pulmonary contusion.
ii. Pulmonary embolus.
iii. Fat embolism syndrome.
iv. Pneumothorax.
v. Aspiration pneumonia.

147 This patient has an occluded left common carotid artery. The artery crosses the thoracic spine from the right, originating from the innominate artery (a 'bovine' arch pattern). The management of blunt injury to the carotid is controversial. In brief, in patients with no neurological deficit, and dissection without occlusion, anticoagulation is appropriate, unless contraindicated. In patients with an early neurological deficit, urgent surgery should be entertained. The majority of neurological deficits are a result of inadequate flow rather than reperfusion injury. In patients with occlusion and fixed deficits, there is no best approach. Ligation and/or anticoagulation are associated with poor outcomes. In many instances the thrombosis extends into the cerebral circulation. Carotid–cavernous fistulae can be managed by embolization. Pseudo-aneurysms can be managed by primary repair, anticoagulation or more complex neurosurgical interventions depending on size and location. Duplex scan will help identify the extent of thrombosis. If the thrombosis extends into the cerebral circulation, anticoagulation and possibly ligation should be considered although there is a significant incidence of late neurological events, presumably from emboli. Other options include subclavian–carotid bypass or direct bypass via sternotomy if the area of thrombosis and/or dissection is limited. Any patient following blunt trauma, with focal CNS changes and negative CT may have sustained a carotid injury and angiography should be considered.

148 **i** and **ii.** Aortic valve incompetence associated with a type A aortic dissection is usually secondary to commissural dissection which can be restored by resuspending the commissures. Patients with aortic annular disease or Marfan's syndrome require aortic valve replacement rather than resuspension and a composite valve graft should be implanted into the aortic root and the coronary ostia anastomosed to the graft. IABP is contraindicated, as it may extend the dissection process; medical treatment using afterload reduction has a much higher mortality over surgical management in type A dissection.

149 **iv.** Pneumothorax occurs in approximately 10–20% of patients with rib fractures who are treated on positive pressure ventilation with PEEP. Some surgeons have recommended prophylactic placement of a chest tube prior to intubation and positive pressure ventilation. This is a life-threatening situation for an ICU patient because the pneumothorax can rapidly become a tension pneumothorax causing haemodynamic compromise. Immediate examination of the chest followed by needle aspiration and chest tube placement on the side where breath sounds are diminished is indicated. High ventilatory pressure and desaturation may be seen in the agitated patient who is biting on the oral endotracheal tube, with right main stem intubations, mucous plugging of the endotracheal tube and bronchospasm. In the unstable patient, one should not wait for a chest radiograph to make the diagnosis of a tension pneumothorax. The other conditions, worsening pulmonary contusion, fat embolism syndrome and aspiration pneumonia, will produce desaturation and increased ventilatory pressure, but the increase in ventilatory pressure occurs over time and is not sudden. Pulmonary embolus produces desaturation but not high ventilatory pressures.

150 A decrease in PCOP is seen with which of the following agents?
i. Adrenaline.
ii. Isoprenaline.
iii. Dobutamine.
iv. Dopamine.
v. Amrinone (aminophylline, milrinone)

151 A 35-year-old, otherwise healthy, woman has a chronic nonproductive cough and recurrent left lower lobe pneumonia leading to abscess formation. What further testing should be done?

152 Which of these incisions are appropriate in a patient with suspected thoracic vascular injuries (152)?

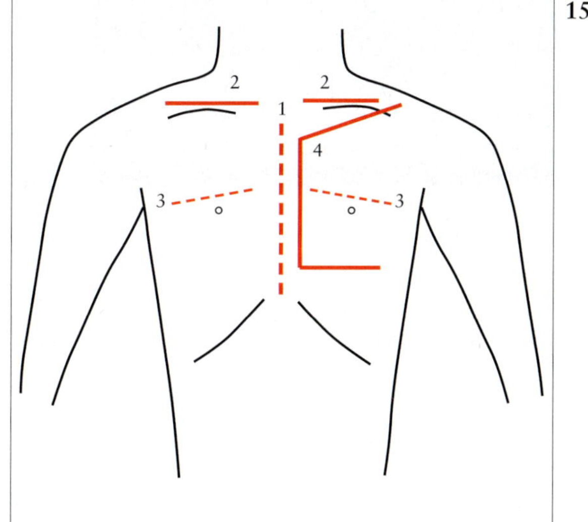

150 Isoprenaline, dobutamine and amrinone all serve to decrease the PCWP. Adrenaline and dopamine, depending on the dosage, either leave the PCWP unchanged or increase it based on the amount of vasoconstriction. Dobutamine and isoprenaline increase CO, decrease SVR and decrease the PCWP. Amrinone, a phosphodextrose inhibitor, is believed to cause vasodilation by increasing intracellular cAMP levels in smooth muscle. The action of amrinone is not related to sympathomimetic stimulation. Similar agents include aminophylline and milrinone.

151

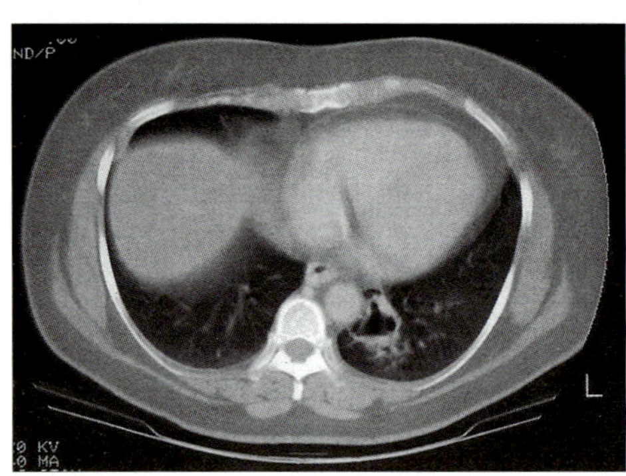

151 A CT scan of the chest (**151**) revealed a left lower lobe abscess with dilated bronchi and the possibility of a systemic artery feeding the lesion. An intralobar sequestration was suspected. Surgical resection was curative. In these congenital lesions, no bronchial communication exists between a pulmonary segment or entire lobe. Usually a systemic artery arising from the abdominal aorta traverses the pulmonary ligament to supply the sequestration. Venous drainage usually occurs to the pulmonary veins but systemic venous connections may be present. Sequestrations can be either extra or intralobar. The extralobar variant is usually asymptomatic and presents as a triangular mass adjacent to the thoracic oesophagus or aorta on the chest radiograph. CT scans are usually diagnostic. Intralobar sequestrations often are found in the lower lungs with a left-sided predominance. Due to collateral ventilation chronic infection and abscess formation can occur. In a newborn, ultrasound may suggest the diagnosis. In older patients a chest CT is the diagnostic mode of choice. Bronchoscopy in obvious cases is not required. Angiography should be considered only if there is a question of the location of the systemic arterial inflow. Any suggestion of oesophageal disorder (reflux, dysphagia, etc) should mandate an oesophagogram. Surgical excision by segmentectomy or lobectomy is curative.

152 All of these approaches can be used. Traditionally, proximal left subclavian injuries are controlled by a left antero-lateral 4th interspace approach, but can be reached by sternotomy with supraclavicular extension.

In patients with gross haemothorax who present in shock and require emergency thoracotomy, tamponade can be achieved by packing the apex of the thorax with an OR gown or sponges. In an unstable patient who can be brought to the OR, sternotomy will allow proximal control to the innominate artery and the left common carotid.

Usually, upon performing sternotomy, the superior mediastinal structures are distorted by haematoma. The pericardium should be opened and the vessels controlled from within this uncontaminated sac. Mobilization of the innominate vein allows access to the superior mediastinal vessels, as well as the trachea.

153 Describe how the steps indicated in the illustration relate to the function of adrenergic and cholinergic receptors (153).

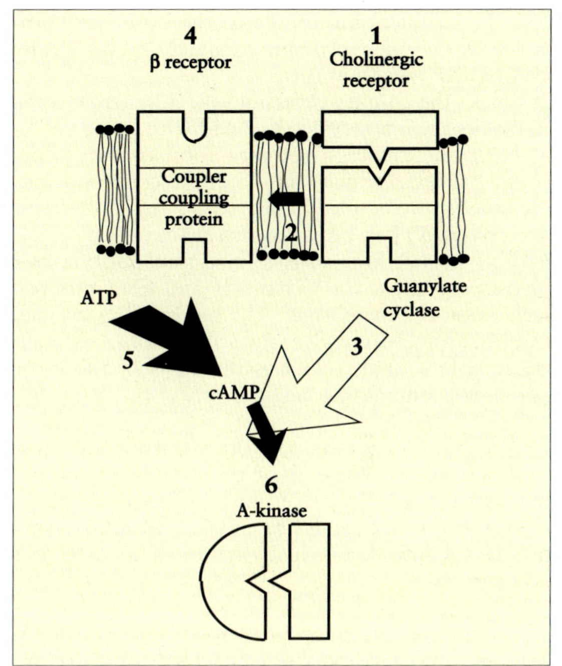

154 What are the Class IV antidysrhythmics?

155 With regard to congenital diaphragmatic herniae, which of the following statement/statements is/are true?:
i. *In utero* surgical correction of the defect is the ideal treatment for the majority of CDHs.
ii. Surgical repair is best done when the infant has been successfully weaned from ECMO/ECLS.
iii. Laparotomy or thoracotomy and urgent surgical repair of the diaphragm should be undertaken regardless of ventilatory status.
iv. ECMO/ECLS should be necessary in less than 50% of CDHs.
v. ECMO/ECLS via either AV or VV cannulation should be instituted when 'conventional ventilation' fails to maintain a postductal $PaO_2 > 100$ torr. $\int 100/13.3$ kPa.

153 1. Acetylcholine binds to the outer protein of the cholinergic receptor. This activates the inner protein, guanylate cyclase, stimulating the conversion of GTP to cyclic GMP, which in turn:
2. Blocks the coupler protein in the adrenergic receptor and
3. Blocks the interaction of cAMP with A-kinase
4. The beta-adrenergic receptor consists of three proteins: an outer receptor; a middle coupler protein which stimulates the conversion of GTP to GMP and also stimulates the inner protein, adenylate cyclase. This protein in turn acts to:
5. Convert ATP to cAMP which then:
6. Activates A-kinase. A-kinase phosphorylates regulatory proteins of the actin-myosin complex, Ca^{2+} channels and Ca^{2+} pumps on the sarcoplasmic reticulum as well as on the membrane. The net result is an increase in intracellular Ca^{2+} concentration, an increased clearance of calcium, and increased sensitivity to calcium by the contractile proteins. This is the basis of the inotropic and chronotropic effects of adrenergic stimulating agents.

154 Class IV agents are the calcium antagonists, which prolong AV nodal conduction and Phase 2 of the action potential. Side effects include heart block, hypotension and negative inotropic effects. These can be prevented by concomitant administration of small amounts of calcium. They can be used for chronic treatment of supraventricular tachyarrhythmias, as well as some of the hypertrophic cardiomyopathies.

155 **ii** and **iv**. Although *in utero* surgery is being done for congenital diaphragmatic herniae in a very few select paediatric and neonatal centres, one must still consider this a relatively experimental treatment and at this time it would not be considered the standard. The majority of congenital diaphragmatic herniae which are symptomatic in the first 24 h of life should be successfully managed with means other than ECMO. Conventional ventilation with NO and other ventilatory modes, such as high frequency oscillatory ventilation, may be all that is required. Where these fail and the child's oxygenation and ventilation are deteriorating, then ECMO should be instituted. Standard protocols are used to decide which infants are appropriately managed this way and it is a decision made jointly with the neonatalogist, cardiologist, surgeon and radiologist. VV or arterial venous bypass may be used; an $aADO_2$ value (>600 mmHg (80.0 kPa)) or an oxygenation index >25 are accurate predictors of mortality and hence the need for ECMO. Because of problems with anticoagulation and haemodynamic instability, procedures are best done following successful weaning from ECMO. Morbidity and mortality are adversely affected by urgent surgical repair of the diaphragm in an unstable child with compromised ventilation and oxygenation.

156 What steps are taken in the initial management of lye ingestion?

157 A newborn infant male weighing 1600 g is diagnosed *in utero* with a space occupying lesion in the right thoracic cavity (157). His twin is normal on ultrasound. He is delivered at 32 weeks' gestation and is tachypnoeic and hypoxic requiring intubation and conventional ventilation with a FiO_2 of 0.75. Management of this infant would ideally be:
i. Immediate AV (or VV) cannulation and placement on ECMO.
ii. Administration of surfactant.
iii. Selective endobronchial intubation and ventilation.
iv. Thoracotomy and lobectomy.
v. High-frequency oscillatory ventilation.

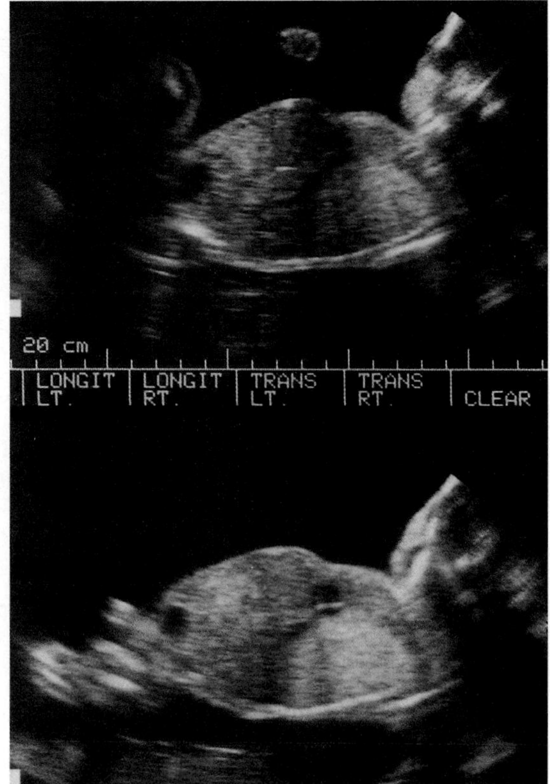

157

158 What are the negative effects of autotransfusion in postoperative cardiac patients?

156 The degree of resuscitation is a function of the cardiopulmonary stability of the patient. In the initial assessment concurrent damage to the lung must be investigated by CXR or bronchoscopy. Parenteral hyperalimentation and broad spectrum antibiotics should be started early. Flexible oesophagoscopy with a paediatric instrument should be performed within the first day to assess the degree and extent of oesophageal and upper GI tract injury. A water-soluble contrast swallow will help to determine whether any perforation has occurred. If this complication is documented, appropriate surgical procedures should be performed to ensure that mediastinal soiling is controlled and drained. CT of the chest and upper abdomen can help assess the degree of injury. Oesophageal strictures that develop may require occasional dilatation. Since oesophageal carcinoma may develop later, long-term surveillance for this complication should be instituted.

157 **ii** and **iv**. The chest radiograph shows a classic picture of a cystic adenomatoid malformation – mixture of solid and cystic elements with mediastinal shift. In addition, the child is premature and there are changes consistent with hyaline membrane disease. The *in utero* ultrasound shows a solid space occupying lesion in the chest.

ECMO is not indicated in this child for a number of reasons: he is too small for successful cannulation and ECMO, but more importantly the usual other conventional means of ventilatory support have not been used. Ideally, administration of surfactant would be the first line of treatment in aims of helping correct the hyaline membrane disease along with conventional ventilation. Once the child is stabilized, removal of the space occupying lesion in the right chest via thoracotomy and lobectomy represents the ideal treatment.

The appearance in the chest radiograph may by confused with a congenital diaphragmatic hernia, but there is no apparent herniation of abdominal viscera and the appearance suggests that both diaphragms are intact. The mediastinal shift and atelectasis are the primary cause of respiratory problems, but very rarely one sees persistent pulmonary hypertension which may ultimately necessitate the use of NO and subsequently ECMO (in an appropriately sized child).

158 Although autotransfusion of shed mediastinal blood may provide a readily available source of blood volume in patients who are actively bleeding postoperatively, several recent studies have suggested that this product may contribute to increased overall bleeding and perhaps increased transfusion requirements. It has been hypothesized that this is related to re-infusion of products of fibrinolysis which are found in high concentrations in this blood. This may subsequently result in stimulation of endothelial tPA production and augmented plasminolysis in the patient. Very consistently, after the re-infusion of these products, the patient's plasma often shows evidence of D-dimer and fibrin degradation products. Therefore, the use of this blood product remains controversial.

159 Discuss indications for CPB to provide non-standard circulatory support.

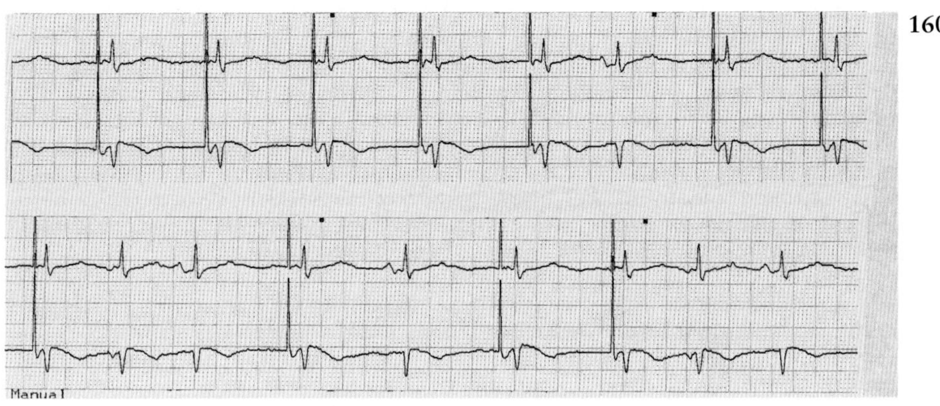

160

160 An ECG for a middle-aged lady with remote CABG and recent repair of ASD. What is the rhythm and the PR interval?

161 A 25-year-old man presents with a gunshot wound to the epigastric area. There is no exit wound. On examination, his blood pressure is 90 mmHg (12.0 kPa) systolic, his heart rate is 110 b.p.m., and his respiratory rate is 20 breaths/min. His breath sounds are equal bilaterally and he has distended neck veins. He is awake and alert with no movement of the lower extremities. Most likely, the aetiology of his hypotension is:
i. Hypovolaemic shock.
ii. Air embolus.
iii. Tension pneumothorax.
iv. Pericardial tamponade.
v. Neurogenic shock.

159 CPB to support patients during repair of congenital and acquired cardiac defects has been performed routinely for many years. Sporadic reports of CPB used outside this purview have appeared over the last three decades. A partial list includes CPB for stabilization of patients with massive pulmonary embolism prior to angiography/and or embolectomy, cardiogenic shock, cardiac arrest from various causes, support of unstable patients during cardiac catheterization, treatment of hypothermia, drug overdoses, trauma, circulatory arrest for CNS aneurysm repair and extraction of renal tumours streaming into the IVC and right heart. Due to the high level of expertise and cost required to implement this technology, limited application has occurred. Parallel evolution of treatment strategies such as thrombolytic therapy, improved inotropic myocardial support and mechanical assist devices have limited the use of CPB in the above settings. Until a clear-cut survival advantage is documented, CPB in these venues will continue to have sporadic application.

160 Atrial pacemaker. Note the large spikes preceding each P wave with appropriate (120 ms) conduction to the ventricles. The sixth atrial complex is spontaneous and sensed appropriately (no pacemaker spike). It was not followed by another spontaneous complex, so pacing automatically resumed.

161 The usual cause of hypotension after penetrating injury is haemorrhagic shock; however, this is inconsistent with this patient's distended neck veins. A large intravascular volume deficit occurs with haemorrhagic shock which should produce flat neck veins. Neurogenic shock is possible in this patient; however, neurogenic shock produces vasodilatation which allows blood to pool in the extremities and is inconsistent with the physical finding of distended neck veins. The complex of hypotension and distended neck veins after trauma is classic for pericardial tamponade, tension pneumothorax, air embolization and myocardial infarction or severe myocardial contusion. Air embolization is unlikely in a spontaneously breathing patient, but does occur when patients are subject to positive pressure ventilation. The finding of bilateral breath sounds being equal is not consistent with the diagnosis of tension pneumothorax. A gunshot wound which can cross or enter the mediastinum with the findings of hypotension and distended neck veins is consistent with pericardial tamponade. Aids to diagnosis of pericardial tamponade in this situation depend upon the perceived stability of the patient. Immediate pericardiocentesis, pericardial window or thoracotomy are performed on patients with impending cardiac arrest from pericardial tamponade. In the more stable patient, a chest radiograph showing air around the heart or a large cardiac shadow may be of assistance. Echocardiography showing increased fluid in the pericardium may also be useful if available.

162 A 65-year-old patient has sudden syncope. Satisfactory CPR is performed. On transport to the hospital the patient is found to be in ventricular tachycardia which is converted with lidocaine (lignocaine). What steps should be taken to work-up this patient?

163 A 53-year-old man presents to the emergency department four days after discharge following an uncomplicated three vessel CABG procedure. His chief complaint is of shaking chills. He has little shortness of breath, his incisional pain has not been increasing and he has no angina. His temperature is 39.3°C. His wounds are healing well without any discharge, his sternum is stable and chest is clear. The chest radiograph shows the same left atelectasis he had at discharge. His urine has no pus cells. His WBC is 23 × 10⁹/l (23,000/mm³). Discuss the differential diagnosis, investigations and management of this patient.

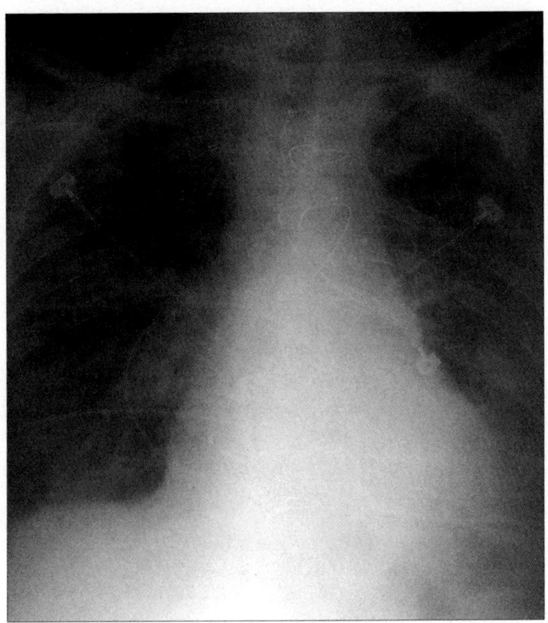

163

164 A 19-year-old man presents with a gunshot wound to the abdomen. His vital signs are heart rate = 120 b.p.m., blood pressure = 96/66 mmHg (12.8/8.8 kPa) and respiratory rate = 22 breaths/min. Two large-bore antecubital IVs are placed and he receives 1 l of Ringer's lactate. His vital signs after fluid are: heart rate = 102 b.p.m., blood pressure = 115/76 mmHg (15.3/10.1 kPa) and respiratory rate = 22 breaths/min. An oximetric Swan–Ganz catheter is inserted which measures his SvO_2 to be 50%. Is this patient in shock?

162 After admission, a monitored environment should be established for documentation of further arrhythmias. Rule out MI and underlying cardiac disease by serial electrocardiograms, cardiac enzymes and catheterization. Electrophysiological studies should be performed to determine whether the ventricular arrhythmia can be suppressed satisfactorily. Indications for implantation of an AICD include documented syncope, cardiac arrest or sustained ventricular tachyarrhythmias without reversible clinical inciting factors, and drug-refractory ventricular tachyarrhythmias documented by electrophysiological testing. Implantation in a heart transplant candidate who has required external countershock for ventricular arrhythmia may increase survival while waiting for a donor organ. The device can be implanted by thoracotomy (sternotomy) or transvenously. The latter has gained popularity since it carries a significantly lower morbidity and mortality. Control of ventricular tachyarrhythmia is similar for both methods of insertion. Deaths following AICD implantation average approximately 2%/year compared to 55% one year survival in similar patients receiving empiric antiarrhythmic therapy. Major long-term complications relate to lead fracture with loss of sensing and/or current delivery, and infection.

163 As with any fever in a postoperative patient, wound infection, both superficial and deep, pneumonia, atelectasis, urinary tract infections and venous thrombosis should be considered. Further investigations should include blood, urine and wound cultures, specifically sternal and substernal aspirates. Radiological investigation of mediastinitis might include CT and WBC scans, although the predictive value is low. Appropriate antibiotics (usually covering *Staphylococcus aureus*) and resuscitative measures must also be addressed. In the absence of another source of infection, a patient who is septic following median sternotomy should have the wound explored. Of note, the sternum is usually unstable with mediastinitis. Mediastinal debridement with insertion of a substernal irrigation system (with or without antibacterial additives) usually will be successful treatment. (Opinion varies as to the advisability of reclosing the incision.) If this method fails, omentopexy, muscle transposition and sternal resection may be necessary. Some advocate these last methods as primary therapy, but most would consider this excessive.

164 Yes. Monitoring of vital signs (heart rate and blood pressure) is standard in the resuscitation of shock patients. Upon normalization of these variables the assumption is that tissue oxygenation is adequate. However, numerous studies have revealed that despite normal vital signs there may be diminished tissue oxygenation. It has been found that 50% of patients resuscitated from shock to normal vital signs had an abnormally low SvO_2 which correlated with the presence of lactic acidosis suggesting oxygen debt. Normal SvO_2 in this patient should be between 65–75%. The low SvO_2 indicates that his tissue beds are extracting oxygen at an abnormally high rate. Hypovolaemic shock models show SvO_2 to be a more sensitive indicator of significant blood loss despite normal vital signs.

165 A 24-year-old man is admitted to the ICU with status asthmaticus. He is intubated and ventilated with assist–control mode; tidal volume 450 ml, rate 8 breaths/min, inspired oxygen 30% and no external PEEP. Appropriate IV sedatives include all of the following, except:
i. Lorazepam.
ii. Ketamine.
iii. Morphine.
iv. Propofol.
v. All the above are acceptable.

166 What are the indications and complications of IABP placement?

167 An 84-year-old man who had descending aortic aneurysm repaired three years earlier presents with shortness of breath on exertion. The chest radiograph and CT scan are shown (**167a, b**). The management should be:
i. Medical management.
ii. Immediate repair of aortic aneurysm under hypothermic arrest.
iii. Mitral valve repair.
iv. Mitral valve repair plus aortic arch surgery.

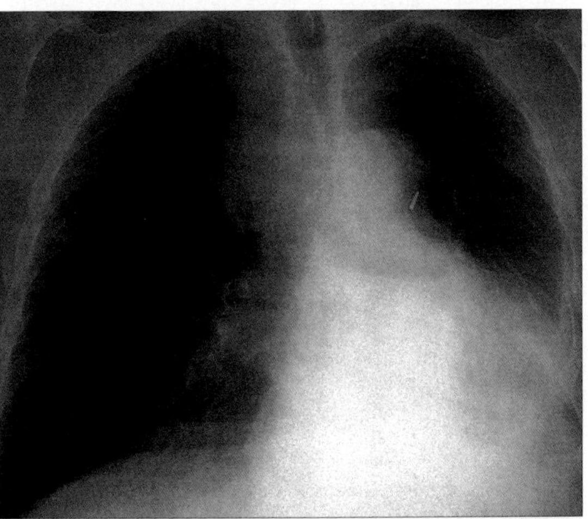

167a

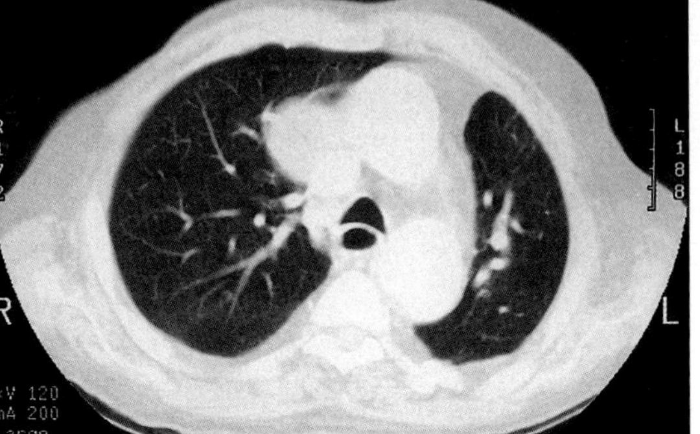

167b

165 v. Patients with status asthmaticus require sedation to allow safe and effective mechanical ventilation. A number of agents have been used successfully, including those listed above. Complications associated with these agents include drug accumulation with lorazepam and prolonged awakening from sedation. The histamine-releasing effects of morphine can be reduced through constant infusion, but ileus is common. Propofol has a rapid onset and is easily titrated to the level of sedation required. Hypertriglyceridaemia may result with high doses. Ketamine provides minimal sedation and analgesia, and may contribute to a delirium-like state.

166 The IABP results in increased diastolic perfusion, and decreased systolic resistance. This in turn results in decreased ventricular wall stress and myocardial demand by up to 20% as well as being associated with an increased CO. Pre-operative and medical indications include: refractory angina; resistant arrhythmias due to ischaemia; complications of infarction including shock, VSD and acute MR; acute myocarditis; as a bridge to transplantation. Postoperative indications include LV failure (MAP <60 mmHg (8.0 kPa), CI <1.8 ml/min/m^2, LA pressure >25 mmHg (3.3 kPa), SVRI >2500 dyne/s/cm^5, all with inotropic support). Contraindications include aortic dissection, aortic insufficiency and severe peripheral vascular disease.

The commonest complication is failure to achieve arterial cannulation and/or inability to pass a wire (5–7%). Intra-operative options range from attempting axillary approaches, transthoracic aortic approaches or even rarely through the abdominal aorta (both needing intra-operative removal). Local complications including false aneurysm, bleeding, vessel thrombosis and threatened limb loss, occur in nearly 10% of cases. Limb ischaemia appears to have been reduced with the introduction of a 'sheathless' catheter. Ideally the ankle-brachial index in the limb used should be >0.6. Heparin may be used, and constant monitoring with Doppler may note early vessel thrombosis. In many situations issues of 'life-vs-limb' may need to be decided. Other vascular complications include aortic rupture or dissection (occurring in 1–2%), or stroke. When placing the IABP, the tip should be kept below the left subclavian and above the renal arteries. Balloon rupture can be caused by a hard plaque, and may be heralded by high pressures. It may be recognized by noting blood in the catheter itself and requires removal, although the catheter can be changed over a guide wire. Systemic complications include thrombocytopenia, possibly related to concomitant heparin administration, and sepsis. Sepsis can be local, if the balloon is placed through a limb of a graft (12% chance) or systemic (1.4%). Appropriate 'sizing' is important; patients <54 kg and 155 cm tall usually require a 34 ml balloon, while larger patients need a 40 ml balloon.

167 i. The optimal approach to the patient would be to pursue medical therapy. Surgery has a high risk due to advanced age, mitral regurgitation and congestive failure. In addition, the mortality and morbidity of a cardiovascular complication might be significant. Long-term survival may not be improved in this instance.

168 Which of the following pharmacological agents have been found to ameliorate cerebral injury associated with CPB?
i. Thiopental.
ii. Heparin.
iii. Prostacyclin.
iv. Nimodipine.

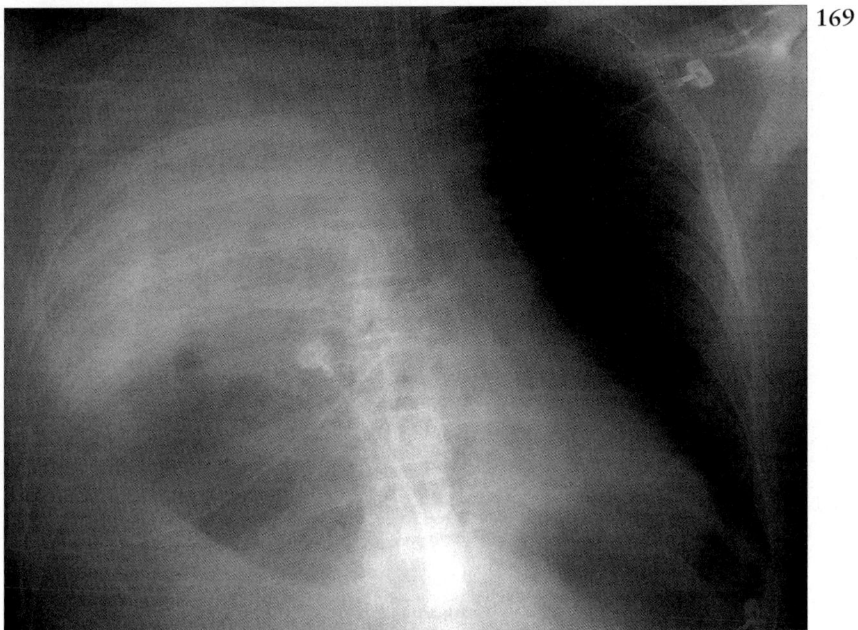

169

169 A pregnant patient develops sudden shortness of breath and right chest pain. A chest radiograph shows a right pleural effusion and a thoracentesis produces blood (169). What are the diagnostic considerations here?

170 With regard to ECMO, which of the following statements are true?:
i. Veno-arterial bypass is preferable to veno-venous bypass when cardiac support is required.
ii. ECMO should not be instituted until conventional and unconventional ventilatory support has been tried for at least 48 h.
iii. Repair of complex 'surgical' lesions may be done on or off ECMO (e.g. CDH, LTE cleft).
iv. There is an absolute time limit of 72 h on ECMO before irreversible complications ensue.
v. A weight of 3 kg or greater is mandatory regarding vessel size for cannulation.

168 i and iv. The brain becomes injured as a result of primary insult due to hypoxia and hypotension. This mechanism of brain injury appears to be similar whether the initiating insult is head injury, cerebral haemorrhage or stroke. Most of the cerebral protectants have been tried at the cellular level to help prevent or modify this effect. Thiopental was shown in one study to significantly reduce persistent neurological defects, but this has not been confirmed in CABG. Calcium channel blockers have been suggested, and of these, nimodipine has been shown to improve postoperative cognitive function six months following surgery.

169 In the absence of trauma or invasive procedures around the thorax, the major consideration in this patient was a ruptured pulmonary arteriovenous malformation. If this lesion is part of the Rendu–Osler–Weber disease (ROWD) a greater number of malformations and complications can be seen. It should be suspected in a patient with solitary or multiple pulmonary nodules when dyspnoea and an unexpectedly low PO_2 are present. Unless part of ROWD, these lesions must be differentiated from other causes of pulmonary nodules. Usually the chest CT is diagnostic showing both pulmonary arterial and venous vessels in association with the nodule. With smaller multiple lesions, pulmonary angiography with embolization can be considered. Larger malformations require surgical excision. Potential complications of untreated lesions include rupture through the visceral pleura with haemothorax, paradoxical embolization and fatigue secondary to the right-to-left shunt. Haemoptysis is rare.

170 i and iii. With regard to time limits and ECMO, there is no hard and fast rule for using conventional ventilatory support before instituting ECMO. A decision to begin ECMO is made on relatively strict criteria based on the alveolar arterial oxygen gradient, oxygenation index and responses of the oxygenation and ventilation to conventional therapy, including NO. There are relative and absolute contraindications, such as severe intracranial haemorrhage, birth weight under 2 kg and severe congenital heart disease. The team of physicians looking after the neonate needs to make a joint decision and cooperation amongst the specialities is mandatory.

Cardiac status must be nearly optimal for successful veno-venous bypass so that veno-arterial bypass is preferred when cardiac function is compromised.

Complex anatomical lesions may be repaired on ECMO – such as repair of a laryngotracheal oesophageal cleft – but where possible one wishes to defer repair until the child has been successfully weaned; for example, congenital diaphragmatic hernia.

171 What is the significance of a prolonged QT interval?

172 A 25-year-old man with a history of intravenous drug use presents with a right groin pulsatile mass, fever and tachycardia. An angiogram shows the following: the Doppler-derived ankle-brachial indices were 0.4/0.4 in the affected leg (**172**). The most appropriate management is:
i. IV antibiotics and observation.
ii. Resection of aneurysm of primary amputation.
iii. Resection and placement of PTFE graft.
iv. Incision and drainage and wound care.
v. Graded compression via ultrasound.
vi. Resection of the infected vessels with ligation and primary bypass with autologous tissue through uninfected tissue planes with muscle flap coverage of the suture lines.

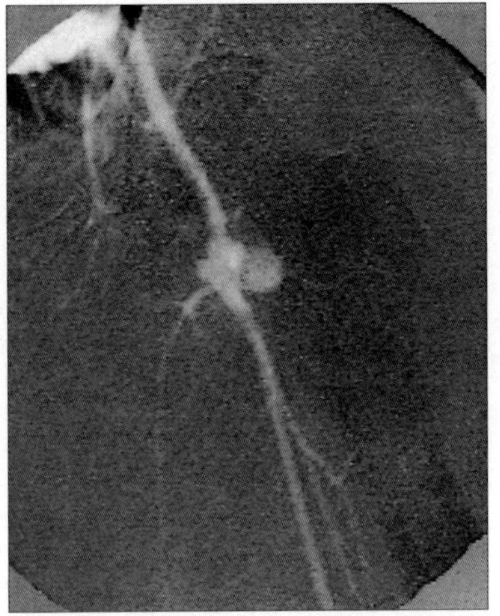

172

173 The best management for a patient with an oesophageal perforation proximal to a chronic hard fibre stricture 3 cm long and 3 cm above the lower oesophageal sphincter in an intrathoracic position is:
i. Thoracotomy and primary repair.
ii. Exclusion and diversion.
iii. Conservative treatment and subsequent dilatation.
iv. Oesophagectomy and immediate or delayed reconstruction.
v. Dilatation and intrathoracic Collis–Nissen repair.

171 The QT interval may be prolonged by ischaemia, anti-arrhythmic agents, and other drugs including Haldol. It may also be congenital (the 'long QT syndrome'). It is measured from the beginning of the QRS complex to the end of the T wave. Marked prolongation of the interval reflects prolonged repolarization, which is associated with an increased risk of polymorphic ventricular tachycardia (Torsades de Points). QT interval is rate dependent, being shorter with faster rates. Thus, a more clinically significant measurement is the 'corrected' QT interval (QTc). This is calculated by the following (in seconds):

$$QTc = (QT\ interval)/(RR\ interval)$$

The upper limit for normal for QTc is 0.44 s.

172 vi. This is an infected pseudoaneurysm and requires surgical debridement to prevent blowout of the artery and/or sepsis. IV antibiotics alone is not adequate treatment. Incision and drainage is extremely dangerous and is often performed due to misdiagnosis. Placement of prosthetic graft is also contraindicated in the infected field. Graded compression is only useful in small injuries such as after cardiac catheterization.

Surgical debridement and coverage of the infected vessel with a muscle flap is necessary. Reconstruction is controversial. Ligation alone is acceptable. However, if faced with a nonviable limb, options such as immediate bypass with autologous conduit or delayed placement of prosthetic graft via uninfected tissue planes are feasible. Routes include femoro-femoral graft crossover and occasionally axillo-femoral bypass. The rate of limb loss with ligation alone depends on the location of the pseudoaneurysm. Ligation of the common iliac artery has an amputation rate of approximately 50%. Ligation of the trifurcation of the common femoral artery/superficial femoral artery/profunda femoral artery has nearly a 67% rate of limb loss.

173 iv. The best management for a patient with a perforation proximal to an undilatable benign structure is resection with either delayed or immediate reconstruction. An intrathoracic fundoplication has a tendency to incarcerate with strangulation at the fundoplication.

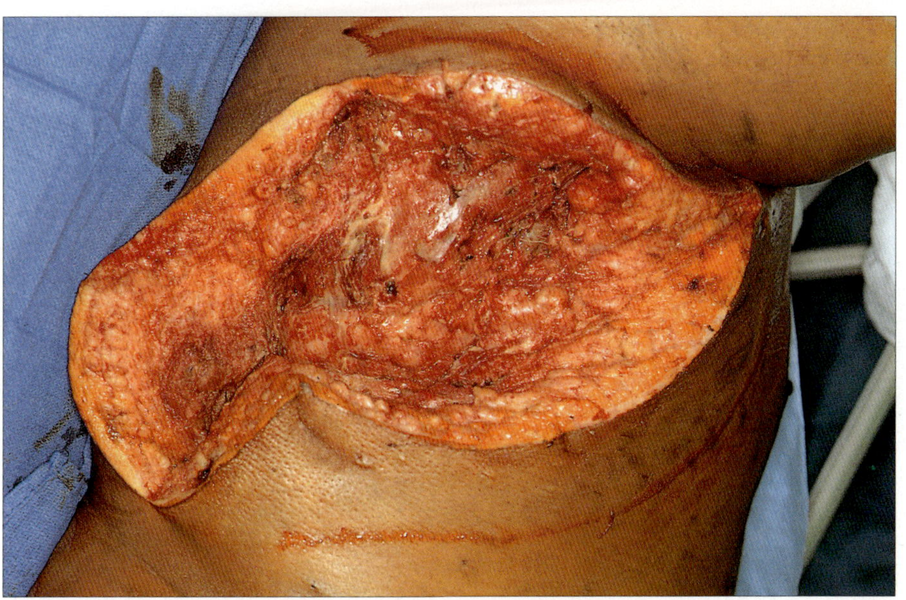

174

174 A 45-year-old obese diabetic patient with sleep apnoea, presented with fever, mild cellulitis and uncontrollable blood sugars. Chest radiograph revealed air in the soft tissues and debridement was carried out. It was found that brawny oedema and pockets of pus, with patchy dead fascia, extended to the rib cage and extensively around the chest cavity (**174**). Briefly discuss necrotizing fasciitis.

175 Discuss the management of haemoptysis.

176 A 45-year-old man is brought to the emergency department in cardiac arrest. CPR is begun and the patient is intubated. An end-tidal CO_2 monitor is attached to the end of the endotracheal tube. Chest compressions are constant at a rate of 72/min and a depth of 5 cm. Ventilation is delivered at a rate of 12/min in a six-compression-to-one-ventilation duty cycle. The end-tidal CO_2 ($PetCO_2$) is 15 mmHg (2.0 kPa). Discuss the end-tidal CO_2 monitoring during cardiac arrest and its predictive value of return of spontaneous circulation.

174 Necrotizing fasciitis presents as an 'iceberg tip' lesion, often with minimal local signs. Inciting factors include diabetes, immune deficiency, local infection, obesity and local trauma. Diagnosis is made by clinical examination, recognizing possible aetiologies and by noting gas in the soft tissue planes. The bacterial pathogens associated with fascitis include beta-haemolytic streptococci, often with staphylococci and/or Gram negatives. Clostridial species are implicated in myonecrosis. The initial management involves aggressive cardiopulmonary/fluid resuscitation, broad spectrum antibiotics and urgent debridement, which is often radical. Wound care includes whirlpool and local debridement. The use of hyperbaric oxygen is controversial, but may play a role following complete debridement.

175 The clinical spectrum of this problem ranges from blood streaked sputum to exsanguinating haemorrhage. Massive haemoptysis is considered when more than 600 ml of blood is coughed per 24 h. In the USA, the most common cause of haemoptysis is bronchitis, and is usually self limiting. Other sources include pulmonary malignancies, granulomatous cavities, bronchiectasis, and rupture of vascular structures into the contiguous lung or tracheobronchial tube. History and physical examination may suggest a source and possibly a site of origin. Chest radiograph and CT depending upon the acuity of the bleeding may further define the source of haemorrhage. If a vascular source is suspected, angiography may define the site. Bronchoscopy should be performed to confirm the side and specific site of bleeding. Placement of the affected side in the down position in conjunction with antitussives may reduce the volume of bleeding. With continued haemoptysis, a bronchial blocker can be placed alongside a bronchoscope and directed into the offending bronchus under direct vision. If this fails, intubation with a double-lumen endotracheal tube should be considered to separate the airways. If bronchial arteriography is available, a search for a vessel supplying the affected area should be made. Embolization may produce temporary control. Surgical exploration should be considered for continued bleeding only when the inciting lesion can be localized.

176 The concentration of expired CO_2 is a result of alveolar ventilation, pulmonary blood flow and production of CO_2. Measurement of end-tidal CO_2 by either infrared absorption or mass-spectrophotometric techniques reflects pulmonary blood flow and CO. After cardiac arrest, a marked decreased of CO and thus pulmonary blood flow occurs. Correspondingly, a decrease in end-tidal CO_2 follows. A prospective clinical study found that end-tidal CO_2 monitoring during CPR could be used as a prognostic indicator of resuscitation and survival. Thirty-five cardiac arrests were studied. Nine patients who were successfully resuscitated had higher average end-tidal CO_2 than those who were not resuscitated (15 mmHg (2.0 kPa) vs. 7 mmHg (0.9 kPa)). No patient with an average end-tidal CO_2 of less than 10 mmHg (1.3 kPa) was resuscitated.

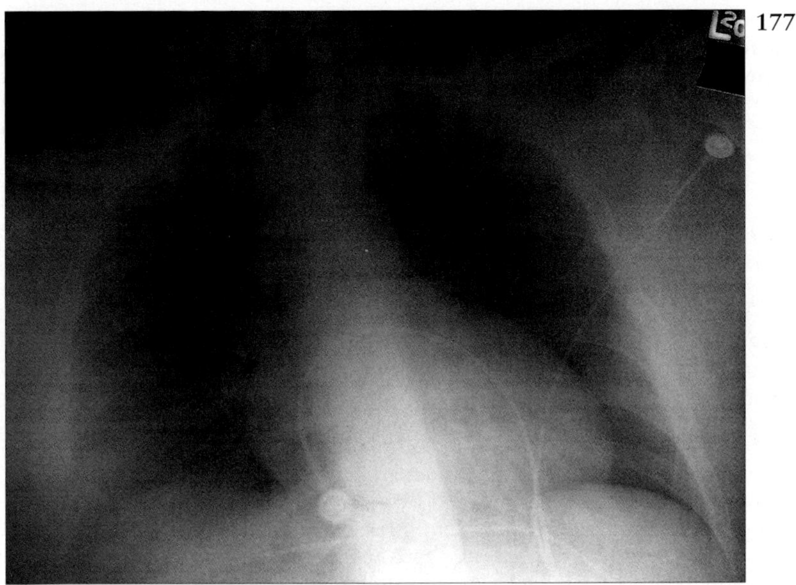

177 This 70-year-old patient presented with hypotension, mild CHF and diffuse abdominal pain. His serum lactate was elevated. He has a history significant for alcohol and tobacco abuse, and two previous MIs. You are asked to rule out intestinal ischaemia. His ECG reveals sinus tachycardia. A chest radiograph is shown (**177**). Discuss your approach.

178 Match the following aetiologies with the correct type of AEF:
i. Thoracic aortic aneurysm.
ii. Repaired thoracic dissection using Dacron graft.
iii. Oesophageal cancer.
iv. Foreign body in the oesophagus.
v. Repaired thoracic aneurysm with PTFE graft.

A. Primary AEF.
B. Secondary AEF.

179 A 72-year-old woman presents with orthopnoea, PND and a history of at least two previous MIs. She is diabetic and is unable to complete a graded exercise test because of shortness of breath. On echocardiography she has an ejection fraction of 18% and severe MR. Coronary angiography demonstrates three vessel coronary artery disease. Thallium scanning shows fixed deficits in the anterior, septal and lateral distributions. What is appropriate management for this patient, and what are the alternatives?

177 This patient probably does have a low flow state involving mesenteric vessels, but it is on the basis of poor cardiac function. In addition, his serum lactate may be chronically elevated because of liver dysfunction. The initial approach in this patient was to optimize his cardiac function. With mild inotropic support and correction of his CHF (in this case dopamine and fursemide), his abdominal pain resolved and his lactic acidosis cleared.

178 i A; ii B; iii A; iv A; v B. Secondary AEF originate from a reconstructed aorta while primary AEF are defined as those involving the untreated aorta. There have been 15 cases of secondary AEF described in the English literature, with only one survivor. Signs and symptoms include haematemesis (80%); signs of infection such as fever, elevated white cell count and/or septic emboli (70%) and thoracic pain (20%).

Primary AEF has been reported in 56 patients, with an overall mortality of 85%. Aetiologies include primary aortic pathology (aneurysm, ulcerated atheromatous plaque, congenital abnormalities of the aorta) in 70%; oesophageal pathology (cancer, infections, ulcer) in 15%; foreign body in the oesophagus in 15%. Presenting symptoms include haematemesis (95%), chest pain (50%), dysphagia (50%) and other symptoms such as abdominal pain and/or septic complications (20%).

Primary AEF is usually approached by extensive debridement, wash out and *in situ* grafting. This approach can be used with secondary AEF if there is not extensive contamination. If there is concern about the degree of infection, complete debridement and rebypass through a clean field should be considered.

179 This woman has three vessel coronary artery disease, severely reduced ventricular function, severe MR and evidence of irreversible ischaemic damage to large areas of myocardium. Options for treatment include medical therapy, angioplasty and surgery. Medical therapy would be directed towards reducing ventricular afterload, limiting salt and water intake, diuresis and, perhaps, anti-anginal therapy, although no ischaemia is demonstrated. Coronary angioplasty is unlikely to be beneficial because of the lack of demonstrated ischaemia. Coronary bypass with mitral valve repair or replacement in patients without evidence of hibernating myocardium and severely depressed ventricular function is very high risk, and functional status in survivors is often disappointing. Cardiac transplantation is not a likely option because of the woman's age and diabetes, both of which are relative contraindications.

In the presence of poor ventricular function (ejection fraction <25%), the presence of angina as the major symptom, or documentation of hibernating myocardium favours proceeding with revascularization. Shortness of breath and the primary complaint argues in favour of medical therapy, particularly when viable myocardium cannot be demonstrated in the areas subtended by diseased arteries.

180 The accompanying chest radiograph was taken in a 29-week gestational baby weighing 800 g. A systolic murmur was heard four days after birth. What is the probable cause?

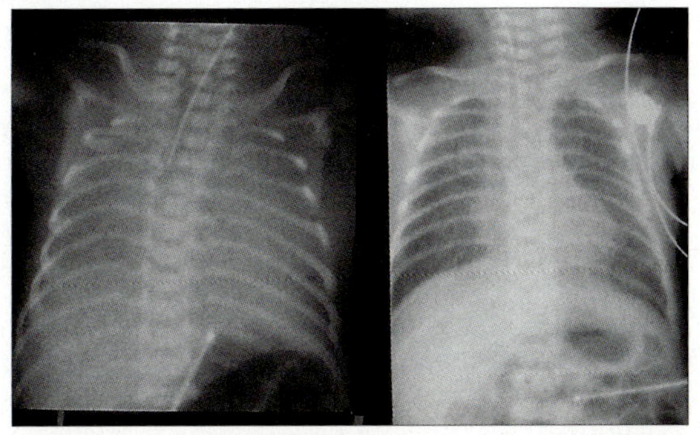

180

181 A 20-year-old man presented with a gun shot wound to the chest. An exploration was performed because of continued bleeding. At surgery, it was found that he sustained injury (181) in the upper one-third of the oesophagus involving slightly less than one-half of the circumference of the oesophagus. The best management is:
i. Oesophagectomy.
ii. Circumferential excision and primary anastomosis.
iii. Lateral repair in two layers and flap reinforcement.
iv. Repair with oesophageal diversion.
v. T-tube drainage.

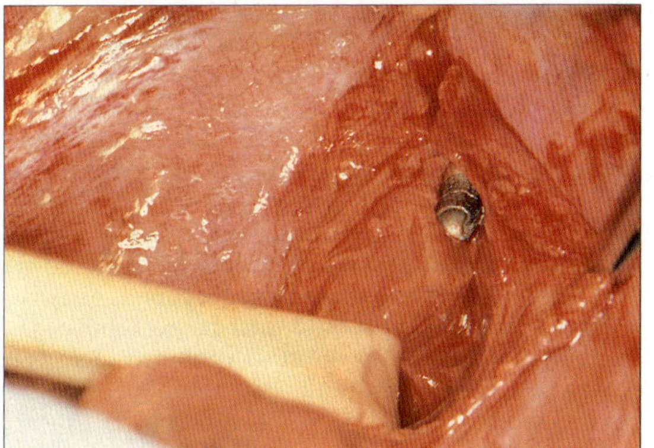

181

182 A 70-year-old man, with a known history of thoracic aneurysm, presents with haemoptysis, chest pain and fevers. Despite this he is clinically stable and chest radiograph is unchanged. Which of the following studies should be performed first?
i. Oesophagogastroscopy.
ii. Upper GI series.
iii. Aortogram.
iv. Indium scan.

180 Due to immature lungs in a pre-term infant, hypoxia often is present. This tends to promote ductal patency. The rate of patency is inversely proportional to the birth weight and gestational age. Due to persistent fetal circulation and high PA pressures, little shunting occurs immediately after delivery. As PA pressures fall, a systolic or continuous murmur develops with associated hyperdynamic precordium and bounding pulses. A chest radiograph will show progressive cardiomegaly with prominent pulmonary vessels and possibly pulmonary oedema. Ultrasonography may show an increased left atrial to aortic ratio associated with ductal flow. Spontaneous closure with fluid restriction may occur. Prostaglandin inhibitors (indomethacin) may promote closure. Often contraindications to this drug's use (azotaemia, bleeding, hyperbilirubinaemia) exist in these small infants. If a brief trial of medical management fails to control the shunt, surgical closure of the ductus should be performed.

181 iii. In acute penetrating injuries to the oesophagus, the best management option is primary repair in two layers with a pleural or muscular viable tissue flap. If greater than 50% of this circumference is lost or if there is concern of major blast injury with tissue necrosis, it may be safer to perform local resection and primary anastomosis. Occasionally drainage is acceptable. Complications of either approach include fistulizations, stricture and leak. The patient should be kept NPO for 5–7 days and have a swallowing study before being allowed to take PO. NG tube is not contraindicated.

182 An unstable patient, with suspected AEF (either primary or secondary), and no contraindications to surgery, should be explored without delay. A stable patient, with a possible AEF should undergo oesophagogastroscopy initially. If that is noncontributory, a CT scan should then be performed. If either are positive, and the patient remains stable, an aortogram is useful to identify the pertinent anatomy. If both are negative, upper GI, indium scan and/or aortogram may be useful. During the work-up the patient's blood pressure should be tightly controlled, as with aortic dissections or aneurysms.

183 A 17-year-old is quadriplegic following a RTA in which he suffered a C5 fracture. He is ventilator dependent and a tracheostomy is placed. You are asked to see him because of recurrent pneumothoraces, 5 on the right, 3 on the left (**183**). Ventilator settings at this point include a pressure support of 10 cm H_2O, CPAP 5 cm H_2O and IMV rate of 8. He has persistent right lower lobe pneumonia. Discuss your approach.

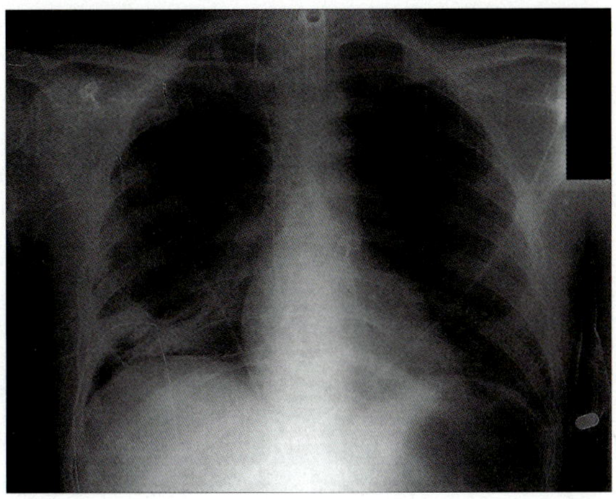

184 A systolic murmur is heard over the primary pulmonic area in a middle-aged woman. The second heart sound has fixed splitting with respirations. A chest radiograph demonstrates an enlarged right ventricle. What is the most likely possibility here?

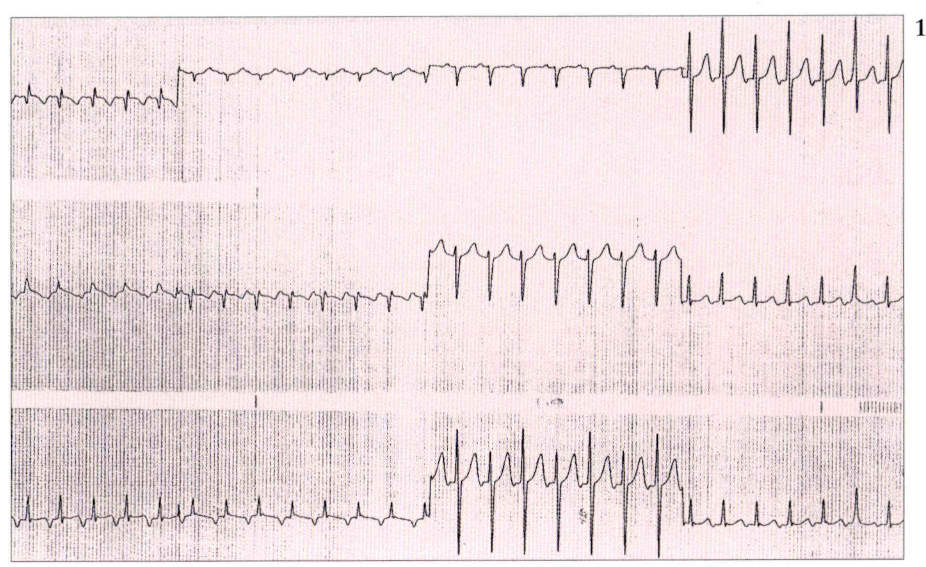

185 An ECG for a 42-year-old woman in good health (**185**). What is the rhythm and the differential diagnosis?

183 This young man may eventually be able to breathe without ventilator support. However, he could not be expected to tolerate a pneumothorax. Because of his age, the approach should be the one with the least recurrence rate. Because of the bilateral problems, both sides need to be addressed. While sternotomy affords a bilateral approach, this is relatively contraindicated because of the pneumonia and the tracheostomy. This latter is a significant risk factor for sternal wound infection. Bilateral submammary incisions were used. It was found that he had large bibasilar blebs, with minimal apical ones. These were resected and pleurectomy performed. Following resection he was ultimately weaned from the ventilator with no further recurrences.

184 Although acquired cardiac lesions may present some of these clinical findings, a congenital ASD is suspect. Those not treated during infancy and childhood may survive many years, but normal life expectancy is not the rule. Often progressive fatigue, atrial arrhythmias, and right heart failure secondary to pulmonary hypertension develop, thus shortening life. In a series of 125 patients over the age of 40 years with ASD treated at Henry Ford Hospital, Detroit, the operative mortality was 4.8%. Preoperatively, 39 of 125 (31.2%) were in NYHA classes 3 and 4, whereas only 8 of 119 (6.7%) were in NYHA 3 and 4 postoperatively. Sudden death, possibly from arrhythmias and cerebrovascular accidents, accounted for the greatest number of late deaths. Closure of the defect in adulthood did not prevent late development of atrial fibrillation. A pulmonary vascular resistance greater than two-thirds systemic values or Eisenmenger's syndrome documented at catheterization contraindicate surgical closure.

185 Supraventricular tachycardia. Note the narrow QRS with alternating amplitude, particularly in V3–V4, which suggests that it is medicated over an accessory pathway. (An ectopic atrial tachycardia would also have to be considered in the differential diagnosis.)

186 The woman in question **185** after administration of IV adenosine. What is the rhythm and the diagnosis?

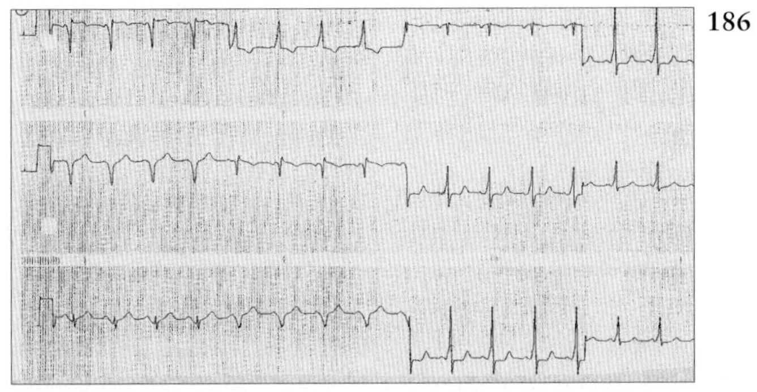

187 ECGs for the same patient as in question **186** one week later (**187a, b**). What procedure has been performed?

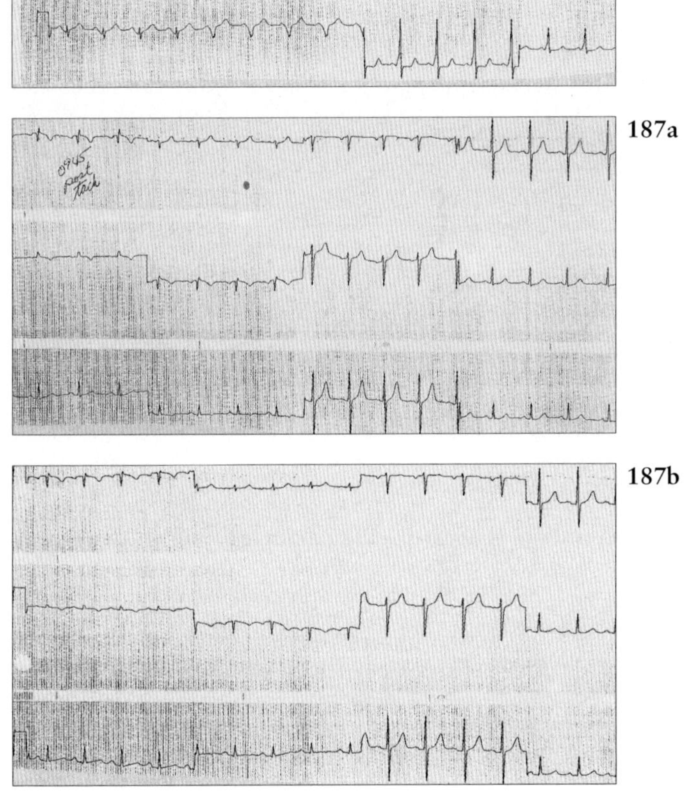

188 What is 'lusitropy'?

189 Discuss the management of oesophageal foreign bodies.

186 WPW is demonstrated with negative 'delta waves' in II, III and AVF and positive 'delta waves' in leads V2–V3 while in normal sinus rhythm. This is suggestive of a posteroseptal accessory pathway.

187 A posteroseptal accessory pathway. Note the flat PR segment and disappearance of delta waves.

188 This is a state of reduced ventricular diastolic compliance, due to congenital heart disease or ischaemia. This results in a chamber that is stiffer, and often has reduced stroke volume. Increased CO can be achieved with careful volume expansion, as well as vasodilation and occasionally 'gentle' use of inotropic agents.

189 Retained oesophageal foreign bodies can occur at any age, but are more common in infants usually less than one year and adults between age 50–60 years. In children they include toys, coins, and small batteries. In adults, sharp bones are the most common variety. Many ingested foreign bodies will pass into the stomach without incarceration. Signs and symptoms of incarceration can include dysphagia, cough, regurgitation, haematemesis, and evidence of perforation. Impaction usually occurs at one of the physiological narrowings: the cricopharyngeus, the aortic arch, and the GE(OG) junction. The majority, however, are seen in the cervical oesophagus. Occurrence at other levels should raise the possibility of intrinsic oesophageal diseases such as strictures, motor disturbances, malignant problems, postoperative stenosis, Schatzki's ring. Impacted meat or repeat foreign bodies in the adult have a high association with intrinsic oesophageal disease. Direct and indirect laryngoscopy should be performed. Occasionally foreign bodies can be visualized in the hypopharynx. A standard CXR and soft tissue view of the neck should be performed to look for mediastinal air and other evidence of oesophageal perforation such as pneumothorax or widened mediastinum. Endoscopy is the treatment of choice for oesophageal foreign bodies. Rigid endoscopy with general anaesthesia permits control of the airway; the rigid scope can be left in place for multiple manoeuvres if necessary. Flexible endoscopy offers less protection for the airway and the extraction rate is not as high as rigid oesophagoscopy. It is important to inspect the entire oesophagus after extraction to rule out perforation and intrinsic disease as an underlying cause. With the rigid oesophagoscope, the extraction rate should approach 99%. There is approximately a 5% chance of perforation. If there is any evidence of perforation, a soluble contrast swallow such as Gastrografin should be performed. Indications for surgical removal of oesophageal foreign bodies include evidence of oesophago-aortic perforation such as a foreign body at the level of the aortic arch associated with haematemesis, significant perforation, and a foreign body too large to be extracted or pushed into the stomach. Since long-term survival with retained foreign body is poor due to complications such as perforation or obstruction, all should be extracted.

190 The incidence of serious ventilator mishaps that are not recognized is very low in an ICU. True or false?

191 A 75-year-old man presents with a bowel obstruction (**191**). Pertinent facts include: mild CHF with an S3 gallop rhythm; MI 2 years previously; Aortic stenosis; 1–2 PVCs/min; chronic renal insufficiency secondary to diabetes. Given these factors, what is the risk of a major cardiac event if:
i. Immediate surgery is required?
ii. Surgery can be delayed to allow optimization?

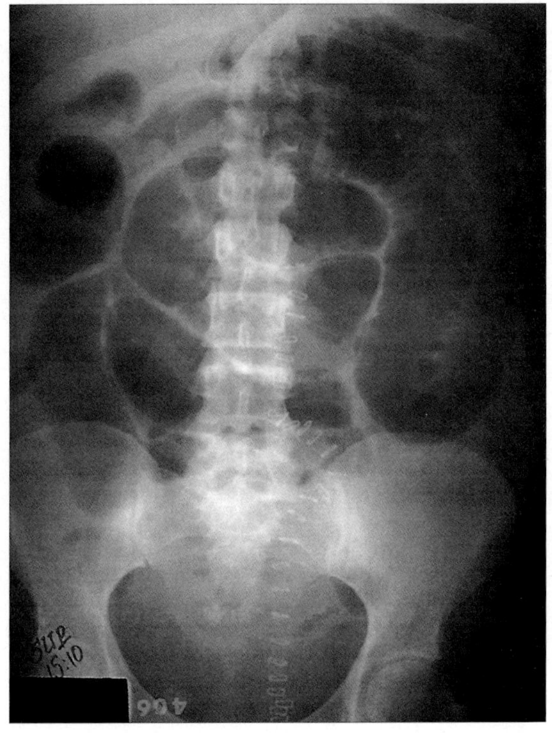

191

192 A 56-year-old woman with a previous anterior myocardial infarction and angina which occurs daily when she carries the laundry from the basement of her house and who is being treated with isosorbide dinitrate, diltiazem, atenolol and ASA, has an angiogram which shows an ejection fraction of 36% and severe proximal stenosis in each of the LAD, circumflex and RCA distributions. Apart from treated hypertension and hypercholesterolaemia, she is otherwise fit. Discuss the benefits and risks of coronary artery bypass surgery in this patient as well as alternative treatments.

190 False. As many as 10% of ICU patients may suffer a ventilator mishap, two-thirds of whom will develop arrhythmias. Serious mishaps (disconnections, pneumo-thorax, plugging, self extubation) have been estimated at one per 20 patient days. The connection between the respiratory problem and arrhythmias is not recognized in the majority of these cases.

191 The risk of cardiac complications developing during non-cardiac procedures can be assessed by the Goldman criteria. In brief, this assigns the following scoring system:

Preoperative condition	Score
S3 gallop/JVD	11
MI <6 months	10
Non-sinus rhythm	7
>5 PVCs	7
Age >70	5
Emergency surgery	4
Intraperitoneal, thoracic or aortic surgery	3
Aortic stenosis	3
Poor medical state	3

Scores	Cardiac complication	Cardiac death
>26	22%	>50%
13–25	11%	2%

If the procedure cannot be put off, this patient has a maximum score of 29. If there is indication that surgical intervention can be postponed to allow 'optimization' with reversal of CHF (possibly with careful diuresis or even use of inotropic agents and pre-operative PA monitoring), the score can be reduced by $(11 + 4) = 15$ points, or now 14.

At present, recurrent MI rates appear to be approximately 15% if a previous MI was less than 3 months prior to surgery, 5–10% if 3–6 months, and at a fixed rate of 3–5% if >6 months.

192 This lady will statistically benefit from CABG over medical therapy with improved life expectancy, less angina, improved exercise tolerance and less require-ment for medication. In addition, there is a reduced risk of myocardial infarction and better preservation of left ventricular function with CABG compared to medical treatment. Risks of CABG include heart attack, heart failure, pulmonary compli-cations, stroke, renal failure, bleeding, infection and other risks common to all opera-tive procedures. Angioplasty may be an acceptable alternative to CABG in selected patients with multivessel disease. It is frequently not technically feasible (perhaps 5–10% of patients with three vessel disease), the rate of reintervention is higher than for comparable CABG patients, as is the incidence of continued angina, and the question of durability is not answered. Angioplasty is however associated with more rapid return to function than CABG, and may be less costly over a period of two years.

193 Briefly discuss PC–IRV.

194 A 35-year-old man is seen in the emergency department following a fight in a bar. This radiograph is obtained (194). His history indicates that he suffered a gun shot wound to the left chest 5 years previously, that was treated with a chest tube only. Is the bullet in the heart? What are the indications for removing foreign objects from the heart in non-acute settings?

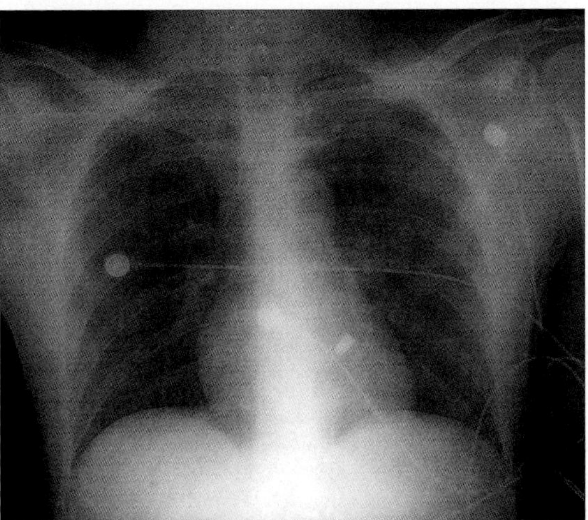

194

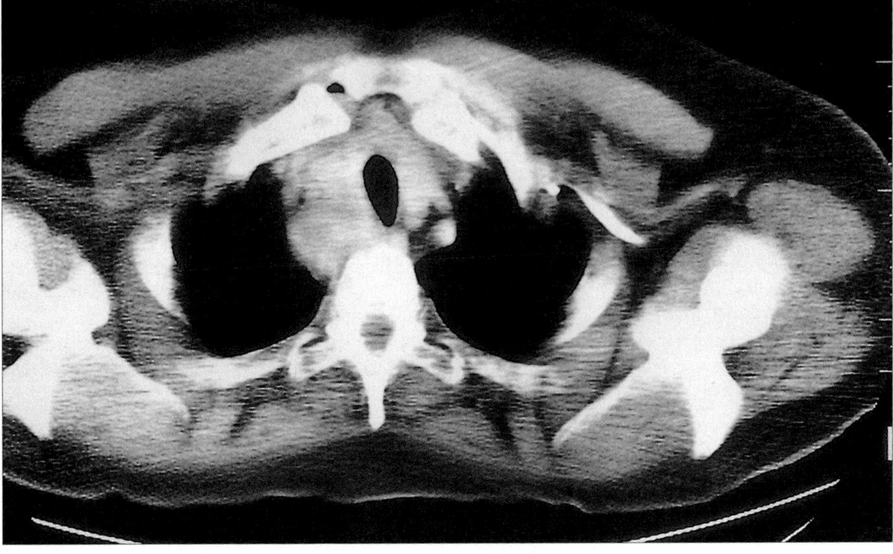

195

195 A 55-year-old man was investigated for change in voice, upper airway stridor and dysphagia. A chest radiograph revealed an antero-superior mediastinal mass. A CT scan is consistent with the lesion being a goiter (195). Discuss the management of this lesion.

193 The reversal of the inspiratory to expiratory time (I>E) is felt to result in a PEEP-like recruitment of alveolar units. The rapid obtaining of respiratory pressure and the subsequent gradual deceleration associated with pressure control waveform appears to result in very even ventilatory distribution and reduction in barotrauma in the more compliant alveolar units. Indications include ARDS (or other restrictive pathology), when PEEP is reaching 15 cm H_2O, PIP >60 mmHg (8.0 kPa). but PaO_2/FiO_2 ratio continues to drop. Currently, it is recognized that these parameters represent late changes, and that PC–IRV should be considered much earlier. Sedation and paralysis are required. Start at FiO_2 of 100%, pressure control at half to two-thirds of PIP, respiratory rate of about 25 breaths/min, I:E of 2:1. One should decrease PEEP to <7 cm H_2O. PaO_2 is regulated by changes in FiO_2 and I:E ratio while $PaCO_2$ is regulated by RR and the pressure control.

Complications include barotrauma and decreased CO, due in part to 'auto' PEEP. It is not uncommon to have to allow a state of 'permissive hypercapnia'.

194 The bullet appears to have sharp edges. Foreign bodies in contact with the heart classically are blurred due to motion artifact. Factors that would tend to support removal of a bullet from the heart include if it is left sided, partially embedded and/or associated with complications (infection, effusion, aneurysm). The depth and site of invasion can be assessed by echo (transthoracic or transoesophageal) or fluoroscopy. Cardiac catheterization is indicated if there is still a concern of intracardiac lesions or associated coronary pathology. Lesions that are asymptomatic, fully imbedded or right sided tend not to need removal. The most appropriate step in evaluating this patient would be to try to compare the current radiograph with the previous one, and obtain a lateral view. Otherwise, no other specific intervention is needed.

195 Intrathoracic goitres are usually benign, usually are extensions of cervical thyroid glands and represent up to 9% of mediastinal masses. True intrathoracic goitres occur only about 0.3% of the time. Indications for removal include risk of malignancy (<5%) and airway compression. Medical management with radioactive iodine is contraindicated, as resultant swelling of the gland can precipitate acute airway obstruction. A similar situation can occur when individuals who live in iodine-depleted areas (such as Kenya) visit a country where iodine is plentiful. After a few days acute haemorrhage can occur into the gland, precipitating swelling and obstructive symptoms.

Because the majority of goitres have cervical blood supply, they can be removed via a cervical approach. The gland most commonly remains to the right and in continuity with the trachea. The recurrent nerve and major vasculature structures can be pushed forward and recurrent nerve injuries occur in up to 10% of cases.

196 Match the drug with the effects:

i. Dopamine
ii. Dobutamine.
iii. Milrinone (aminophylline, amrinone).

A. Increases coronary blood flow.
B. Dose-dependent effects.
C. Associated with thrombocytopenia.
D. Peripheral vasoconstrictor.
E. No increase in myocardial O_2 consumption.
F. Increases cAMP.
G. Releases endogenous adrenaline and noradrenaline.

197 A schematic of events which occur during a cardiac cycle is shown (**197**). Answer the following:
i. What do the a, c, x, v and y in the venous pressures represent?
ii. What do the four heart sounds represent?
iii. What is meant by an 'opening snap' and 'ejection click'?

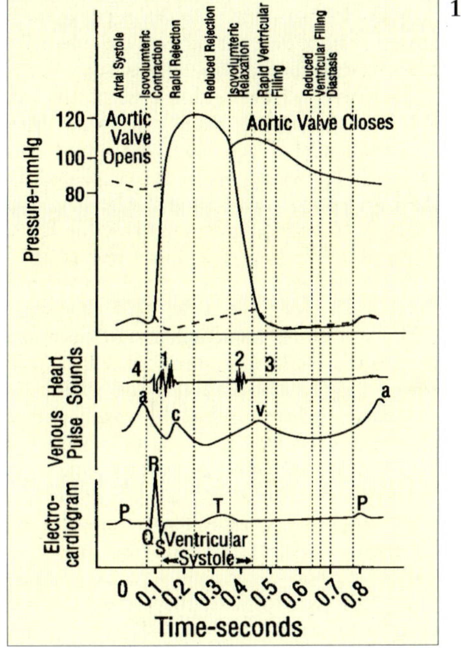

198 A 68-year-old man suffers a non-Q myocardial infarction following a laparotomy for perforated duodenal ulcer. His recovery is complicated by mild CHF but not by angina. Echocardiography reveals his ejection fraction to be 25% with generalized hypokinesia, antero-apical myocardial thinning and mild MR. Coronary angiography shows: 95% stenosis of the LAD with 80% narrowing of the first diagonal, 90% narrowing of the proximal circumflex and occlusion of his RCA which reconstitutes well distally. Thallium scanning shows large areas of reversible ischaemia in the lateral and inferior distributions. Discuss the indications, timing and results of CABG in this patient.

196 Dopamine is an endogenous catecholamine which is an immediate precursor of noradrenaline. It releases both adrenaline and noradrenaline. The effects of dopamine are dose related. In low doses, it acts on the dopaminergic receptors causing vasodilation. A high dose acts as a vasoconstrictor in the arterial and venous capillary beds. Dobutamine stimulates the β_1-, β_2-, and α-receptors. Dobutamine increases myocardial oxygen consumption, but it also increases myocardial oxygen delivery by increasing coronary blood flow as a result of decreased coronary vascular resistance. Milrinone, although a positive inotropic agent, is not related to sympathomimetic stimulation. This drug acts by increasing levels of cAMP and the modulation of intracellular calcium. Milrinone increases cardiac output; however, myocardial oxygen consumption is not increased.

197 The a wave occurs as the atrium contracts. The c wave is a result of mitral/tricuspid closure. The v wave represents filling of the atria while the AV valves are closed. The x descent reflects downward pulling of septum during systole while the y descent reflects diastolic emptying.

The first heart sound is created by the rapid tightening of chordae resulting in AV valve closure. More rapid closure, with tachycardia or shortened PR interval, results in a louder S1. Decreased ventricular contractility or increased PR interval leads to a quieter S1. The second heart sound (S2) is caused by the closure of the pulmonary (PA) and aortic (Ao) valves. The PA S2 tends to occur later as a result of lower pulmonary resistance and slightly later RV contraction. Increased resistance (e.g. valvar stenosis) will delay S2. The third heart sound (S3) is also called ventricular gallop. This sound occurs when a volume of inflow enters the ventricle during diastole and 'hits' the ventricular wall. This therefore implies either an excessively large volume, such as in mitral insufficiency, or decreased compliance of the ventricle, such as occurs in chronic ischaemic states or CHF. It can be normal in athletes. The fourth heart sound (S4) is also called atrial gallop. This results when a vigorous atrial ejection results in inflow volume hitting a stiff ventricle. This can occur with hypertrophic cardiomyopathy, aortic or pulmonary stenosis. A summation gallop represents a fusion of both S3 and S4 and implies volume overload.

Fusion of valvar or subvalvar structures will result in loud opening of valves. Ejection click is created by the opening of a diseased pulmonary or aortic valve, while an opening snap is caused by the opening of diseased AV valves.

198 This patient with three vessel coronary artery disease, severely reduced ventricular dysfunction and evidence of hibernating or stunned myocardium will undoubtedly benefit from CABG when compared to medical therapy. Optimal timing of surgery is less certain, although non-Q infarction with demonstrable ischaemia is an unstable situation with 5% hospital mortality. Death is more likely when angina is present and still more likely when angina occurs in the presence of ECG changes. Thus CABG is recommended during the same hospital admission. Results of surgery in this situation depend upon comorbidities as well as the patient's age, but most would quote an operative mortality of approximately 3–5%. Survival at 5 years should be >90% (compared to 60% for medical therapy). The effect of CABG on ventricular function in this situation is unpredictable, although very likely this patient would experience substantial improvement in ventricular function and perhaps complete resolution of his MR.

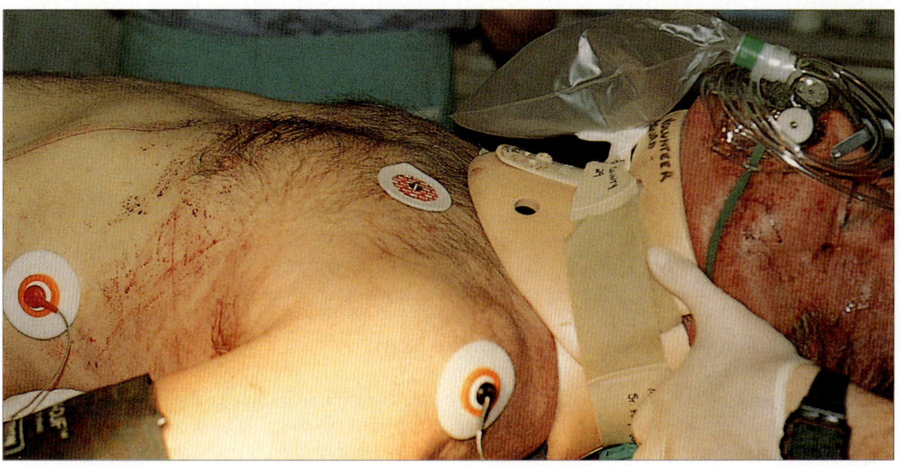

199

199 This patient was found under a car which had apparently collapsed on him while he was working on it (**199**). He is mildly confused, has cyanosis of his face and upper extremities, is stridorous and has petechiae. Discuss the management of this patient.

200 A 33-year-old, 85 kg man with end-stage cardiomyopathy and type B positive blood has been accepted for cardiac transplantation. He is CMV negative. A donor heart from a 30-year-old, 45 kg woman, type O negative blood, following a severe head injury is available. The donor is CMV positive. Which of the following statements is/are true?
i. The donor heart should be refused because of size mismatch between donor and recipient.
ii. The donor heart should be refused because of CMV positive donor.
iii. The recipient could receive a heterotopic heart transplant.
iv. Severe head injury in the donor makes the heart unsuitable for transplantation.

201 A 50-year-old man was admitted following a RTA, in which he was an unrestrained driver. Despite several litres of fluid resuscitation, he remained hypotensive, with a systolic blood pressure of 70–80 mmHg (9.3–10.7 kPa). His heart rate ranged from 80–110 b.p.m. Initial chest radiograph revealed some mediastinal widening and blunting of the aortic knob. ECG revealed only nonspecific ST wave changes. CPK-MB fractions were normal. A transthoracic echocardiogram was reported as normal.
i. What aetiologies can explain these vital signs?
ii. What is the pathophysiology of myocardial contusion?
iii. Discuss the management of myocardial contusion associated with cardiogenic shock.
iv. What is the role of CPK-MB fractions in evaluating this injury?

199 Traumatic asphyxia refers to a syndrome of sudden compression of the superior vena cava and its tributaries. This acute venous hypertension leads to haemorrhage and swelling. Significant airway and cerebral oedema can occur. Initial airway management includes supplying humidified oxygen, upright position and possibly steroids and/or racemic adrenaline. Early intubation may be needed. Extreme cases of cerebral oedema may required intracranial monitoring.

200 i and iii. There is a 40 kg weight mismatch between the donor and the recipient and the donor heart should generally not be accepted. Though it is possible that a heterotopic heart transplant can be performed, the results of these are not satisfactory and is not commonly performed. CMV mismatch is not a contraindication for transplant and severe head injury in the donor does not make a heart unsuitable for transplantation unless there is trauma to the heart.

201 i. The initial evaluation of multiply injured patients includes ATLS principles. A DPL will quickly rule out significant free intraperitoneal bleeding. This patient, however, does not have a tachycardia that is in proportion to his hypotension, raising the possibility of a neurogenic/spinal injury, myocardial contusion or a history of taking medications like beta-blockers. This patient had a negative DPL. There was no evidence of neurogenic shock, as initial spine radiographs were negative and there was no peripheral vasodilation. Despite normal transthoracic echo, which is often inaccurate in this setting, myocardial contusion must be strongly suspected (as this patient was subsequently proven to have).
ii. Myocardial contusion is characterized by patchy and irregular myocardial cell necrosis. The right ventricle is most frequently involved, although the left ventricle can also be affected. The associated cardiac dysfunction and dysrhythmias have been related to transitory redistribution of coronary flow which can be aggravated by hypovolaemia.
iii. Low CO can affect as many as 65% of patients with clinically documented blunt myocardial injury. Cardiogenic shock can be present in 10% of cases. Management includes careful fluid administration, inotropic support and occasionally IABP. Because of right ventricular dysfunction, cardiac function can be further compromised by increasing PEEP. Treatment aimed at decreasing pulmonary hypertension, such as hyperventilation, lower PEEP and pulmonary vasodilators such as dobutamine should be considered. Before placing an IABP, an injury to the thoracic aorta must be ruled out. Other options include percutaneous bypass with heparin-bonded pumps.
iv. Serum CPK-MBs do not appear useful in predicting which patients are at risk of developing complications and are probably not a cost-effective test. Troponin I assays may prove more specific and useful.

202 Discuss the initial evaluation of a neonate with suspected congenital heart disease.

203 Discuss the management of this patient who presented with haemoptysis (**203**).

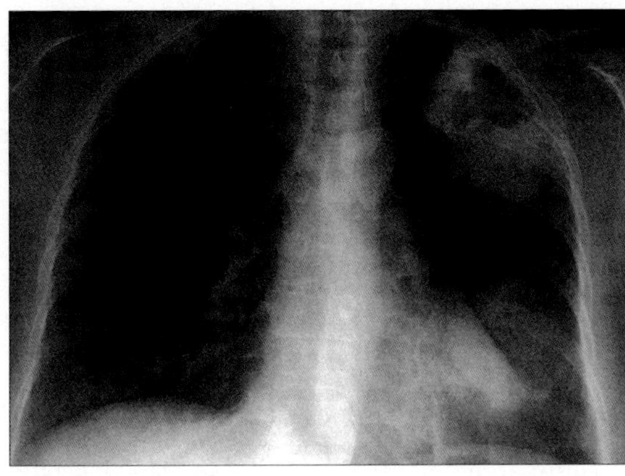

204 A patient is sent to you with a diagnosis of aortic insufficiency. There is a long history of cardiac murmur, no shortness of breath on exertion, no arrhythmias and good exercise tolerance. Discuss the management of this patient with respect to investigations and intervention.

205 This patient presented with a gunshot wound to the chest (**205**). The next step is:
i. Lung resection.
ii. Antibiotics.
iii. Percutaneous drainage.
iv. Bronchoscopy.
v. Observation and pulmonary toilet.

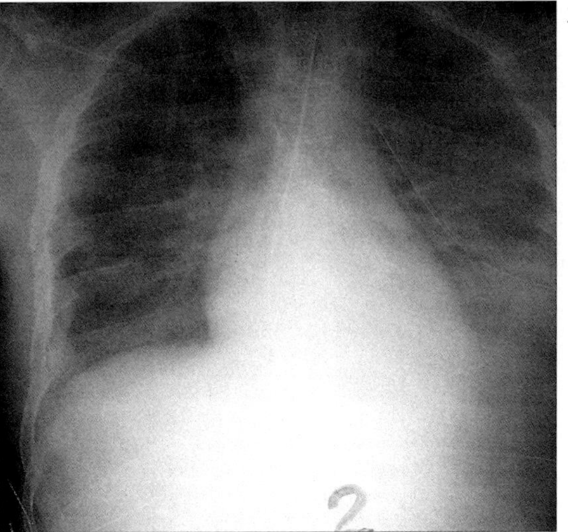

202 The initial approach includes a thorough examination to rule out noncardiac causes of decompensation as well as assessing the severity of the patient's condition. Neonatal sepsis can present as shock or cyanosis, as can noncardiac thoracic emergencies including diaphragmatic hernia, aspiration, etc. Initial work-up includes a chest radiograph, ABG and CBC. Subsequently, echocardiography is extremely important. If the patient is in shock, or severely cyanosed, trial of prostaglandin to maintain ductal patency may be lifesaving and allow time to correct metabolic derangements. Cardiac catheterization may be performed in some settings to better understand the pathophysiology, to identify key anatomic features (e.g. coronary anatomy for TOF if considering repair), and/or to treat the patient (e.g. septostomy).

203 Three clinical forms of aspergillosis involve the lung: aspergillar bronchitis, invasive pulmonary aspergillosis, and aspergilloma ('fungus ball'). Allergic aspergillar bronchitis is not a surgical problem. IPA usually occurs in immunocompromised patients and is usually treated with an antifungal agent such a Amphotericin B. However, the pneumonic process may progress to lung infarction with cavitation. This may produce initial massive haemoptysis which can be life-threatening. Although controversial, resection of localized cavitary IPA has been accomplished, if pulmonary function permits, with relatively low mortality and recurrence. The more common aspergilloma which often colonises a persisting cavity from old tuberculosis, bullous disease, or sarcoidosis may bleed in approximately half the cases. In those with limited pulmonary function, bronchial artery embolization, if possible, can be considered. Transcutaneous puncture of the cavity with instillation of Amphotericin B may resolve the bleeding problem temporarily. It can be repeated as necessary. Cavernostomy or transfer of muscle flaps into the cavity may avoid resection in those with limited pulmonary function. Definitive therapy involves resection of the cavity. Most can be treated with a combination of lobectomy and systemic Amphotericin B with low morbidity and mortality.

204 Tachycardia, ventricular dilatation and eccentric hypertrophy allow long-term compensation in aortic regurgitation. Prior to developing symptoms, evidence of reduced systolic function may be detected, characterized by systolic and diastolic ventricular dilation and reduction of ejection fraction with exercise. If such evidence of asymptomatic decompensation is present, surgery should be strongly considered. Presence of symptoms indicates surgery. Investigation of this patient should include echocardiography, some form of exercise ventriculography and, perhaps, cardiac catheterization (mostly for indentification of coronary artery abnormalities, and only if surgery is contemplated, as most information needed may be obtained by non-invasive methods).

205 v. This patient has a pulmonary haematoma. The management of haematoma is conservative. Strict observation is needed to try to identify complications including empyema, rebleeding of the haemothorax, fibrothorax, abscess formation and haemoptysis. The work-up may require a CT scan for confirmation. Often these lesions decompress endobronchially, but if persistent or troublesome haemoptysis or other complications occur, embolization or surgery should be considered.

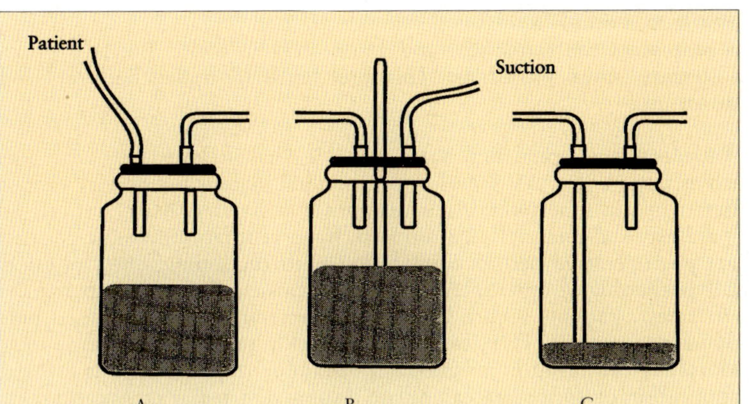

206 In what order should the chest tubes be set up (206)?
i. Patient–A–B–C–wall suction.
ii. Patient–A–C–B–wall suction.
iii. Patient–C–B–A–suction.
iv. Patient–B–A–C–suction.

207 Which of the following therapeutic interventions carries the highest risk of being potentially fatal to a neonate who has undergone correction of anomalous pulmonary venous drainage in the immediate postoperative period?
i. Administration of morphine sulphate.
ii. Endotracheal suctioning.
iii. Giving a fluid bolus 20 ml/kg.
iv. Applying ice bags to the child's forehead.

208 On the third day following an uncomplicated right pneumonectomy, progressive shortness of breath develops. What are the potential causes?

206 ii. Bottle A is simply a fluid collection device and is placed closest to the patient. Bottle C represents the water seal and comes next in order. Bottle B provides the 'Suction Pressure' and is placed last. This three bottle set-up has been replaced by the pleurovac set-up.

207 ii. Patients whose congenital heart pathology has included excessive pulmonary flow, such as large VSDs, AV septal defects and anomalous pulmonary venous drainage, suffer from extreme pulmonary vasomotor reactivity. Many centres advocate routine paralysis and fentanyl sedation with hyperventilation in such patients in the immediate postoperative period. Stimulation with suctioning, chest physiotherapy, acidosis, hypothermia or other interventions can cause pulmonary hypertensive crisis, leading to arrest. Patients whose CHD was characterized by decreased pulmonary flow (pulmonary stenosis, TOF, etc) tend to develop pulmonary oedema much more easily. Morphine can result in a significant histamine response with tachycardia. The simple application of an ice bag can ablate a supraventricular tachycardia. However, it could also result in some pulmonary stimulation if the child is not deeply sedated. Finally, avoidance of acidosis and hypothermia is useful in reducing the risk of crisis.

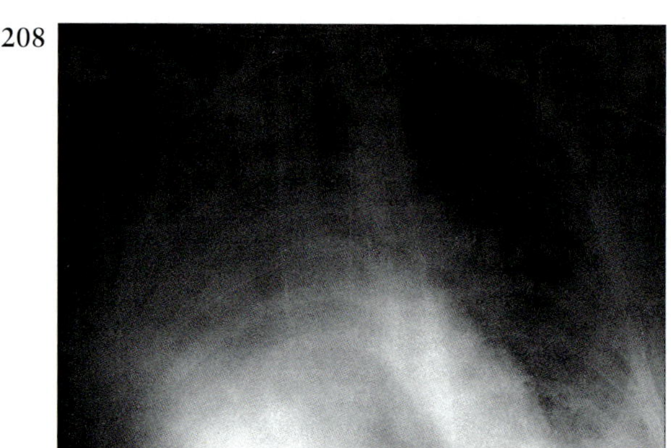

208 Atelectasis should be readily apparent on a chest radiograph (**208**). Pneumonia, although unusual at this time in the postoperative period, should also have a characteristic radiograph and clinical presentation. Pulmonary embolism can be ruled out by VQ scan or angiogram. Bronchial stump dehiscence is usually associated with significant subcutaneous emphysema and coughing of fluid from the operated hemithorax. Progressive dyspnoea, arterial desaturation, and an interstitial oedema pattern on the chest radiograph should suggest post pneumonectomy pulmonary oedema. This usually develops following right pneumonectomy but can rarely be seen following left-sided surgery. It usually develops when the perioperative fluid infusion exceeds 3 l. Its presentation often occurs several days following operation. Treatment depends on the degree of respiratory embarrassment. Supplemental oxygen with vigorous diuresis should be tried. Further deterioration mandates intubation with mechanical ventilation and positive end expiratory pressure. IV fluids should be kept to a minimal rate to allow organ perfusion. If the patient is hypervolaemic, diuretics should be used. Antibiotics and steroids do not seem to affect the outcome. Mortality for this complication averages 50%. Prevention centres around restricting fluid in the immediate perioperative period.

209 You are asked to see an elderly patient in the respiratory ICU who on plain film has developed 'free air'. History included right lower lobectomy for cancer the previous week and steroid-dependent COPD. He has been on the ventilator since surgery, and has been tolerating tube feeds. CT scans have been obtained (**209a, b**). On examination you note subcutaneous emphysema and minimal abdominal tenderness. Does he require immediate surgery?

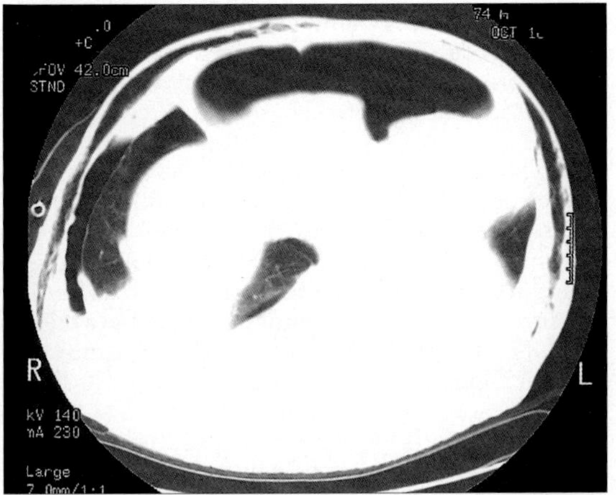

209a

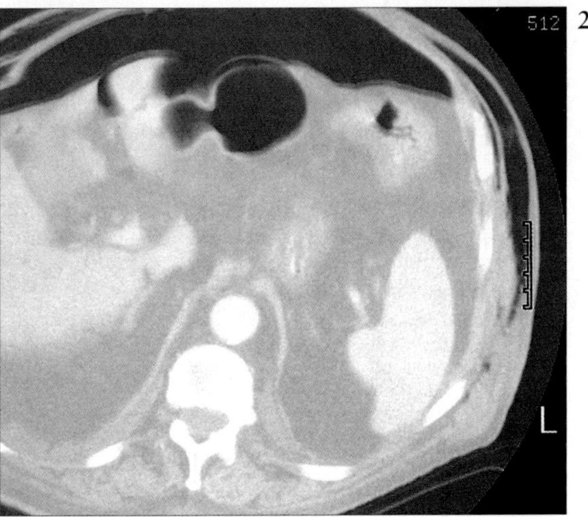

209b

210 What is 'permissive hypercapnia'?

211 Describe a clinical classification of congenital heart disease.

212 What is ICAM and what is its importance?

209 This patient is unlikely to have a free visceral perforation if he continues to tolerate feeds. While this does not entirely rule the possibility out, the CT demonstrates properitoneal air extending down from a residual pneumothorax in the chest without leak of contrast. He should receive another chest tube.

210 This is an approach to ventilation in severe respiratory failure, such as ARDS, where the $PaCO_2$ is allowed to rise to levels of 60 mmHg (8.0 kPa) or even higher. The resultant acidosis may be managed with sodium bicarbonate or THAM if clinically indicated or if pH <7.20 ($[H^+]$ >60). The advantage is felt to be that oxygenation can continue, while avoiding the significant negative impact of higher airway pressures required for ventilation (i.e. blowing off CO_2). Although relatively new, there is suggestive evidence that there may be a survival advantage with this approach in ARDS.

211 In general, congenital heart disease can be categorized according to the dominant findings. Lesions whose predominant feature is cyanosis include:

- PFC.
- TGA.
- Hypoplastic right heart syndromes.
- TOF.

The diagnosis of PFC may be suggested by a history of perinatal trauma/stress (aspiration, maternal infection, etc). Unlike the patient with PFC, a patient with TGA tends not to be extremely distressed, apart from a baseline increased respiratory rate. Patients with pulmonary causes of cyanosis, on FiO_2 of 1.0 should respond by raising the PO_2 to above 100 mmHg (13.3 kPa) (hyperoxia challenge). Hypoplastic right heart syndromes include tricuspid atresia, pulmonary atresia and pulmonary stenosis. TOF may present early in life with severe cyanosis or later with gradual cyanosis depending on the degree of infundibular obstruction.

Lesions presenting with the predominant picture of pulmonary oedema include:

- Truncus arteriosus.
- VSD.
- Total anomalous pulmonary venous connection.

These conditions often have cyanosis as a mild feature.

Lesions presenting as systemic shock include left-sided obstructive lesions such as:

- Aortic stenosis.
- HLHS.
- Co-arctation of the aorta.
- Origin of left coronary from PA.

212 ICAM-1 is an endothelial cell adhesion molecule for PMNs. Its importance is that it plays a key role in the development of multiple organ failure, including ARDS, as the adherence of PMNs to the vessel walls is the basis of the subsequent inflammatory response. Aetiologies include haemorrhagic shock and sepsis. The presence of the soluble form of ICAM has indeed been correlated with the development of MOF.

213 A young man had suffered a through and through gunshot wound to the right chest, requiring surgical repair of the middle and lower lobes. He subsequently developed pneumonia, and elevated PA pressures. Shortly after obtaining this radiograph (**213**), it was noted that he began to desaturate. Despite increasing inspired oxygen from 45 to 100%, there was little increase in saturation. Airway pressure only rose minimally. What might be the cause?

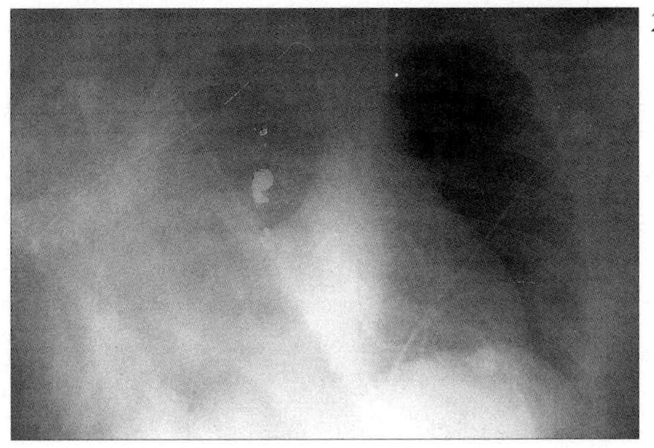

214 This 47-year-old woman presents with complaints of upper abdominal and substernal chest pain, vomiting and melena. Her chest radiograph demonstrates elevation of the left diaphragm. Her upper GI is shown (**214**). Briefly discuss:
i. The pathophysiology of diaphragmatic paralysis and eventration.
ii. GI complications of diaphragmatic paralysis.

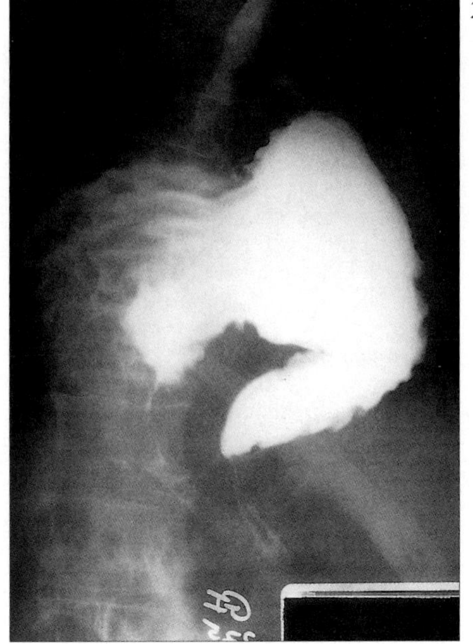

215 Briefly discuss the embryological difference between Primum and Secundum ASDs.

213 Although any number of aetiologies for increased A–a gradient and shunt can be described, failure to respond to the 'hyperoxia' challenge suggests an intracardiac lesion. This patient had a patent foramen ovale which was 'opened' due to increased right-sided pressures. If his hypoxia had continued, he might have needed surgical closure. However, within 24 h he responded to antibiotics and diuresis. This may also occur following pneumonectomy.

214 i. Diaphragmatic eventration and paralysis are related phenomena. Both may be acquired or congenital, partial or complete, temporary or permanent. Paralysis may be due to central pathology (upper motor neurone) or peripheral (lower motor neurone). Acquired aetiologies include birth trauma, neck or thoracic surgery. The commonest adult form is viral. Unilateral paralysis results in a 25% reduction in FRC which is well tolerated by adults but not neonates. Indications for surgery in neonates and infants include ventilatory dependency, repeated pulmonary infections, failure to thrive, feeding difficulties or a large eventration in an asymptomatic child. Plication does not appear to prevent the subsequent return of function. In adults, work-up includes fluoroscopy and the 'sniff test'. Most appear to have involvement of lower motor neurones and only 9% of the idiopathic will return to normal. In patients who have not undergone surgery or suffered other trauma, neck and mediastinal tumours should be ruled out. Asymptomatic patients do not require surgery.
ii. Eventrated or paralysed diaphragm on the left can result in distortion of gastric attachments leading to gastric volvulus, which should be considered a surgical disease. Often, plication is all that is needed, but evidence should be sought for para-oesophageal hernia and/or reflux that might necessitate antireflux procedures concomitantly.

215 The formation of the atrial septum involves the descent from the roof of the infolding atrial chambers of the septum primum to meet the endocardial cushions, which come in 'laterally'. If there is a deficiency in the endocardial cushions, a Primum ASD results. Because the mitral and tricuspid apparatus derive some elements form these same cushions, Primum ASDs are associated with mitral insufficiency, and are really a form of AV septal defect. They are associated with 'cleft' mitral valves and the degree of mitral valve dysfunction is often the most important prognostic indicator. Repair can be complicated by pulmonary hypertension and the need to repair the mitral valve.

If the septum meets the endocardial cushion, but is deficient at the 'top' a Secundum ASD is formed. This has much less physiological significance.

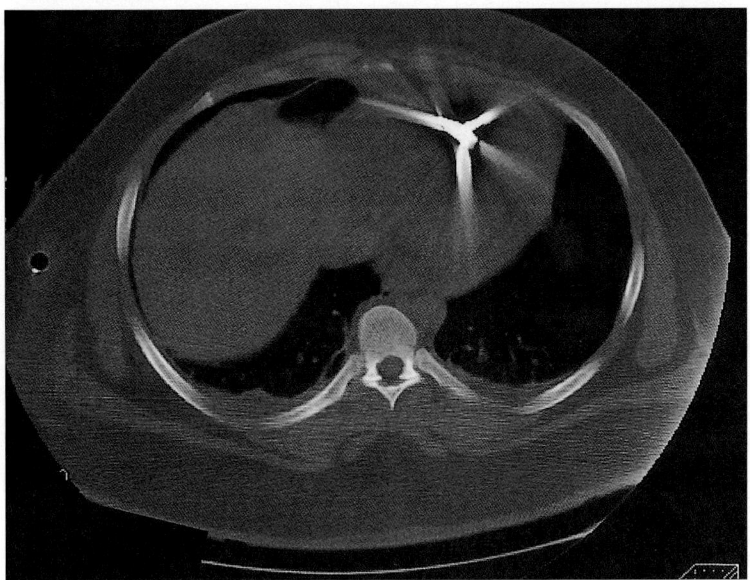
216

216 This patient, with a history of renal failure requiring dialysis, had suffered a gunshot wound to the lower right chest and abdomen (including liver) 7 days previously. He now presents with shortness of breath, jugular venous distention, and low grade fever. Chest radiograph suggested infiltrate and cardiac enlargement. A CT scan, obtained to evaluate chest and upper abdomen, is presented (**216**). The next best step is:
i. Thorascopic pericardiectomy.
ii. Subxiphoid drainage.
iii. Pericardiocentesis.
iv. Pericardial resection through anterolateral thoracotomy.
v. Any of the above.

217 If a neonate needed a pulmonary artery band, what difference would there be in the degree of banding between a child with cyanotic congenital heart disease as opposed to one without cyanosis?

218 A 56-year-old man presents with a second episode this week of temporary left-sided weakness. He has had two previous MIs and continues to have CCS class 3 angina. Carotid Doppler examination shows an occluded left internal carotid artery with a 90% stenosis of the right internal carotid. Discuss the further evaluation and management of this patient.

216 v. This patient has significant clinical signs and symptoms of pericardial effusion, the aetiology of which includes trauma, uraemia and/or infection.

Effusive pericardial effusions and pericarditis have the following differential: idiopathic; infectious (viral, TB, bacterial, parasitic), neoplastic (primary/secondary), metabolic (uraemic, myxoedema), connective tissue disorders, post injury (trauma, myocardial infarction, surgical), or drug induced (procainamide, hydralazine, penicillin, INH, quinidine). The bacterial cause of pericarditis is related to *Staphylococcus aureus*.

Uraemic pericarditis occurs in 20% of acute and 50% of chronic renal failure cases. Effusions have the following incidence: 1–3% after MI, 5–50% after cardiac surgery, 20% after acute renal failure and 50% in cases of chronic renal failure. Indications for surgery include recurrent effusions with evidence of tamponade, evidence of infection or inability to rule out cancer. Uraemic pericarditis results in clinically significant effusions in 15% of cases. Treatment options include increasing cycle of dialysis, the use of NSAIDs, or drainage of the pericardium. The combination of NSAIDs and dialysis can pose significant risk of bleeding.

Drainage can be done by needle aspiration. Surgical approaches include: subxiphoid drainage, thorascopic resection and drainage, or thoracotomy and pericardiectomy.

217 Because cyanotic heart diseases rely more on pulmonary 'mixing' and flow, the initial band determination, using the 'Toronto' formula is 24 mm + 1 mm/kg as opposed to 20 mm + 1 mm/kg for noncyanotic heart disease. At the time of surgery, response can also be measured by measuring systemic saturations, looking at the atrial appendage to detect colour changes and systemic pressures. The goal is to decrease PA pressures by 30–50% of systemic pressures, ideally without decreasing systemic saturation. Often systolic pressure increases 10–15 mmHg (1.3–2.0 kPa).

218 The simultaneous presence of symptomatic cerebrovascular disease and coronary artery disease presents a therapeutic dilemma: should one lesion be addressed prior to the other or both together? If the carotid disease is tacked first, the patient may suffer an MI and if the coronaries are addressed first, a stroke might occur. If addressed simultaneously, the morbidity of each procedure is combined. A reasonable approach is that the most symptomatic lesion should be addressed first, and if both are very symptomatic, then a combined procedure should be planned.

This patient requires angiography of his cerebral and coronary circulations, as well as an assessment of ventricular function and general medical status. As both lesions are very symptomatic, a simultaneous operation should be planned. A sensible operative approach is to first open the chest and make all the precardiopulmonary bypass preparations including harvesting conduit, opening the pericardium and placement of aortic and atrial pursestring sutures. After this the carotid endarterectomy may be done (probably using a shunt in this instance), instituting CPB only in the event of haemodynamic instability. Another approach would be to institute CPB with hypothermia prior to performing the endarterectomy followed by coronary artery bypass during the rewarming period. No randomized data exist to further clarify this controversial area.

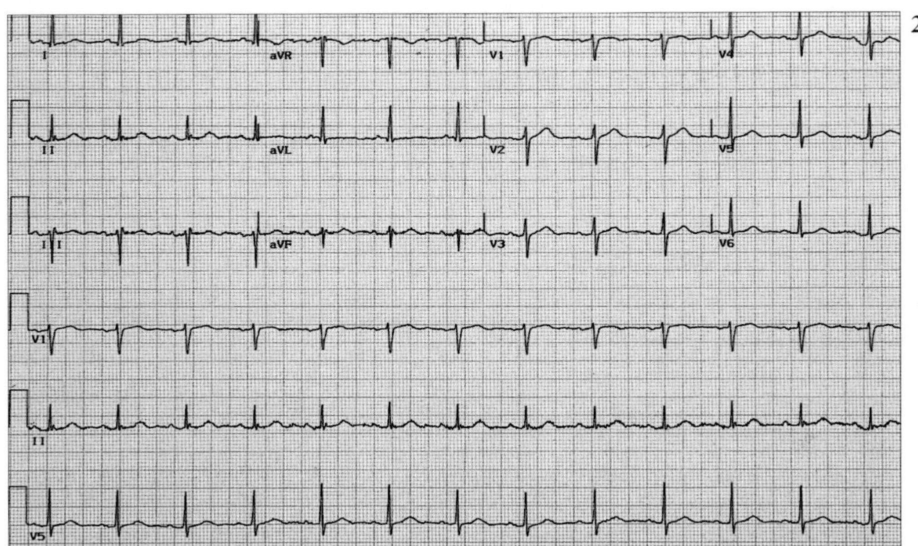

219 A 65-year-old man is admitted to the emergency department after a RTA. He complains only of mild chest wall bruising and tenderness. His ECG is shown (**219**). Past history is significant for a three vessel bypass five years previously. He has not had angina since then. The most appropriate next step in management is:
i. Transthoracic echo.
ii. Serial CPK-MB levels.
iii. Admission to a telemetry unit for overnight observation.
iv. Repeat ECG in 4 h and obtain previous ECGs for comparison.
v. Cardiac catheterization.

220 Discuss the role of the 'Z' score in planning repair of pulmonary atresia.

221 A 72-year-old man presents with CCS class 4 angina and a recent history of syncope. Investigations reveal three vessel coronary artery disease with a mean aortic valve gradient of 65 mmHg (8.7 kPa), a valve area of 0.72 cm², and reduced ventricular function with an ejection fraction of 32%. His haemoglobin is 134 g/l and creatinine is 187 mmol/l (3.95 mg/dl). He is a Jehovah's Witness. Discuss methods of blood conservation which may and may not be employed in this patient.

219 Blunt myocardial injury, often referred to as contusion, represents a spectrum of injuries from asymptomatic to frank rupture. The diagnosis and management is confounded by a lack of clear data regarding the significance of this injury. Most efforts are now directed to detecting which patients are at risk of developing complications, including life-threatening arrhythmias or cardiogenic shock. In this regard, the use of CPK-MBs do not appear useful, and probably result in a significant number of unwarranted admissions and tying up of telemetry units.

In patients who have evidence of low CO, valve injury, arrhythmias or new cardiac symptoms, the most appropriate management is admission to a telemetry unit, serial ECGs and early echo. Transoesophageal echoes are probably more accurate than transthoracic. Patients with unchanged ECGs and no new cardiac symptoms can be observed in a nontelemetry setting and asymptomatic patients with repeated normal ECG after 4 h need not be admitted in many cases. Patients with significant pelvic or craniofacial injuries are at increased risk of developing complications and should be monitored more closely. Tropinin I may prove to be of predictive value.

220 The ability to perform a complete repair in the setting of pulmonary atresia is closely linked to the size and development of the right ventricular chamber. The smaller the chamber, the less likely there will be adequate function, and in addition, the more likely there will be sinusoids which preclude decompression of the ventricle. The size of the ventricle correlates with the development of the tricuspid valve. The Z score refers to the number of standard deviations from the mean that the tricuspid valve is smaller than. If the score is >-1.5, biventricular repair is likely possible. If it is <-4, biventricular repair will probably never be possible, and palliative shunting aiming ultimately for Fontan is usually recommended. Sizes between -4 and -1.5 require individualization. Some patients can be managed by combining valvotomy and shunting as an initial procedure, followed by staged biventricular repair at a later date.

221 Jehovah's Witnesses refuse to accept homologous blood product transfusions and many, though not all, will not allow their own blood to be returned to them if it has been sequestered away from their circulation. This man's acute presentation limits the usefulness of erythropoetin and iron administration, which must be used in more chronic situations to raise haemoglobin levels preoperatively. Autologous predonation is not an option. ASA, heparin and other antithrombotic medications might be discontinued, although the safety of this is questionable given the acute symptoms. Operative measures, such as acute normovolaemic heamodilution and cell saving, should be discussed with the patient, as many will agree to the use of these. Medications, such as aminocaproic acid, tranaxaemic acid, aprotinin (with some reservations when renal function is compromised) and DDAVP, should be employed, as these may limit non-surgical bleeding. Careful attention to surgical haemostasis, as in all operations, is mandatory in cases such as this. There is limited experience with heparin-coated cardiopulmonary bypass equipment, but its use has reduced blood loss, when used with low heparin doses. Postoperatively, re-infusion of shed mediastinal blood is usually not agreed to, but its use should be explored with the patient. Laboratory testing should be limited to an absolute minimum.

Despite all these precautions, mortality risk with surgery is greater for these patients than for those who will accept homologous transfusions, and this requires clear documentation in the consent process.

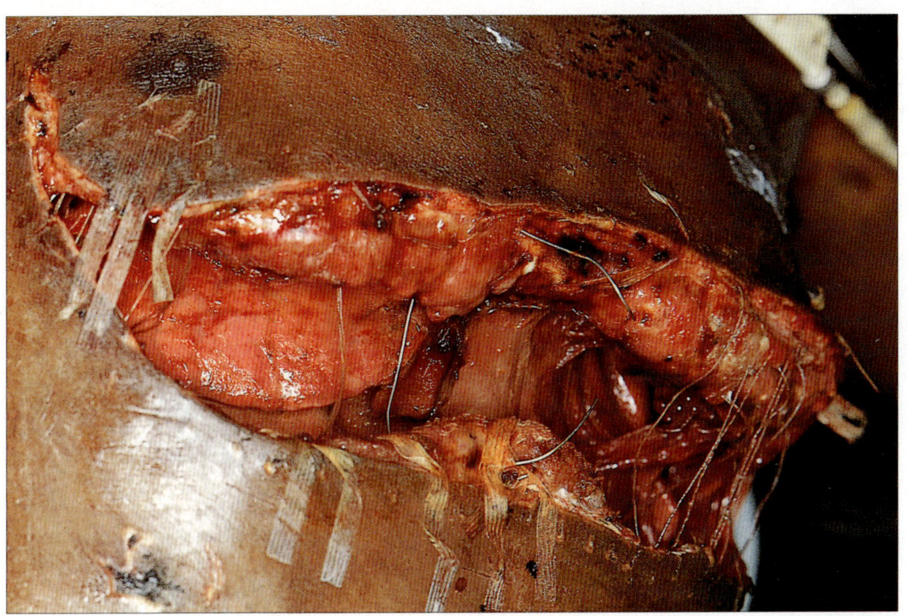

222

222 This 23-year-old man had suffered a gun shot to the right chest (**222**). He arrested *en route* to the emergency department and underwent left thoracotomy and aortic occlusion. A small right atrial injury necessitated extension across the sternum with right thoracotomy. Two days later he was found to have dehiscence of the entire incision. Discuss:
i. The role of emergency thoracotomy in penetrating trauma.
ii. The management of this complication.

223 What criteria can be used to determine whether a neonate with TGA is ready for an arterial switch operation?

224 A 45-year-old man presents to the emergency room with acute occlusion of right femoral artery. He had mechanical mitral valve replacement two years earlier. Echocardiogram shows clot on the mitral prosthesis. The definitive treatment should include which of the following?
i. Administration of thrombolytic drugs.
ii. Heparinization.
iii. Femoral embolectomy followed by mitral valve replacement.
iv. IVC filter.

222 i. Resuscitative thoracotomy, also called EBT, has a few select indications. Patients who may benefit from EBT include those with solitary penetrating chest trauma, who have signs of life on arrival or, if are in arrest, have been intubated in the field and who have evidence of cardiac activity. Patients who present in arrest following blunt trauma, who have extrathoracic trauma or who have no detectable vital signs at the scene should rarely, if ever, undergo thoracotomy.

The approach to penetrating chest trauma and suspected cardiac injuries, can vary depending on where it is performed. In the OR, the best approach is median sternotomy, which requires extension in only 2% of cases for additional exposure. Antero-lateral thoracotomy is most commonly used in the emergency department and requires extension in up to 20% of cases.

Patients who present with right-sided chest trauma and require urgent thoracotomy can be approached via right or left thoracotomy. Proponents of left thoracotomy feel that better CPR can be maintained and that the aorta should be occluded. Proponents of the right-side-first approach feel that right-sided injuries are more easily approached, that CPR can be performed through the right chest, and that aortic occlusion has a minor role in EBT. Whatever one's views, a chest tube should be placed in the unopened hemithorax.
ii. Chest wall dehiscence occurs as a consequence of technical errors, division of the internal mammary artery, infection and tension. Early dehiscence implies poor surgical technique. Once it occurs, debridement of non-viable and infected tissue and closure with the use of omentum or muscle flaps is usually required.

223 Of patients with TGA, 70% have an intact ventricular septum, and thus very early on the morphological left ventricle loses its 'conditioning' provided by the neonatal elevation in PVR, and thus its ability to function as a systemic ventricle. Most centres would try to perform arterial switches before 2 weeks of age for this reason. The ability of the morphological LV to face systemic pressure requirements can be determined by an absence of RV septal bulging into the LV, the thickness of the posterior LV wall, and/or a pressure ratio of LV to RV of >0.6. If these criteria are not met, but there are no other contraindications to ASO, a temporary PA band can be placed to allow development of LV hypertrophy. This may lead to significant improvement within a week.

224 iii. Distal embolization is a known complication of mechanical mitral valve replacement, especially if the coagulation status is not adequate (recommended PT INR 3.5–4). Thrombolytic therapy has been tried with indifferent results. Heparinization is used initially to prevent further thrombosis and/or emboli. IVC filter is not indicated in arterial occlusion. Surgery is the preferred approach.

225 What is the significance of minimally displaced sternal fractures?

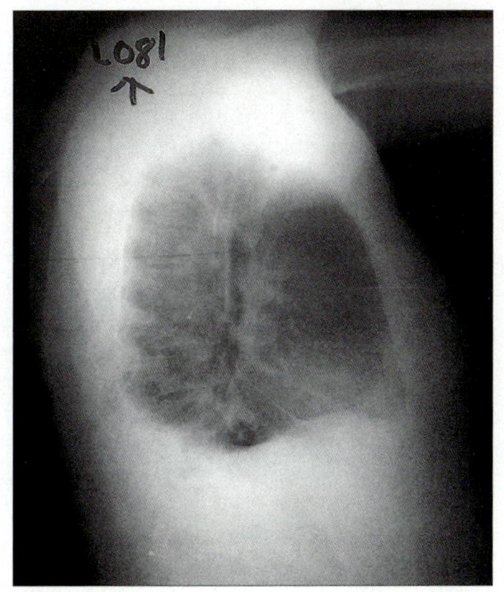

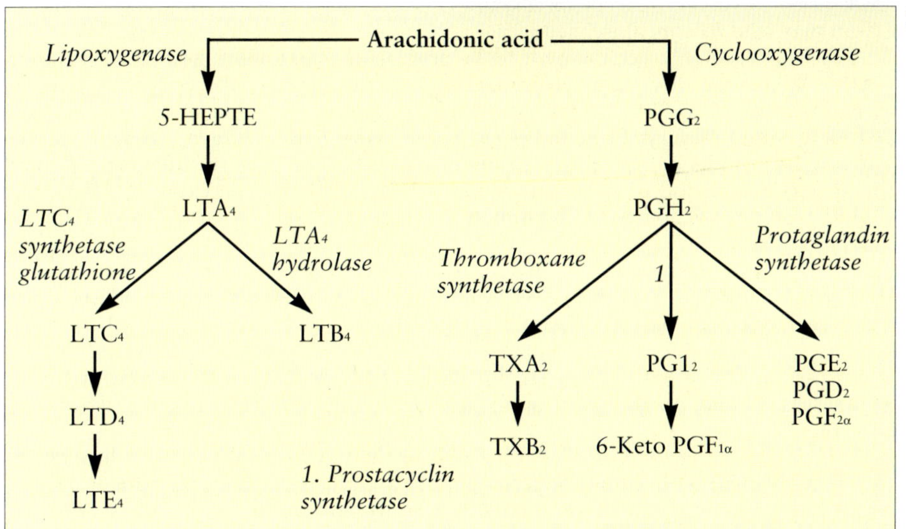

226 A 55-year-old man with chronic stable angina and triple vessel disease, undergoes routine CABG. Discuss the rationale of the perioperative administration of ASA in patients with coronary artery disease.

227 Discuss the perioperative management of patients with anterosuperior mediastinal masses.

225 Sternal fractures alone are uncomplicated, if painful, injuries. Indications for fixation or debridement include the development of sternal infection, severe pain or gross instability preventing proper pulmonary toilet, or need for thoracotomy for another reason. Although there is concern for possible blunt myocardial or aortic injury, in the absence of suggestive findings (ECG changes, widened mediastinum, etc) these possible injuries probably do not require extensive work-up. This patient ultimately developed a significant haematoma which became infected, requiring sternal debridement.

226 Undoubtedly, ASA, the most popular oral anti-platelet medication, has been proven to be extremely effective in the treatment of coronary artery disease. Notably, in patients with stable and unstable angina, the cessation of therapy with this drug may be followed by the abrupt acceleration of symptoms due to the formation of intracoronary platelet thrombi.

Unfortunately, like all anti-thrombotic medications, ASA may contribute to excessive bleeding. Due to the irreversible nature of the platelet enzyme inhibition, this acquired coagulopathy will persist for the duration of the platelet's life (7 days). In patients undergoing cardiac surgery, excessive bleeding was confirmed in prospective randomized studies in which ASA was not stopped preoperatively. As a result of this, most surgical groups stop their patients from taking ASA at least one week prior to surgery, except in cases of unstable angina, when stopping the medication may lead to critical ischaemia.

ASA has repeatedly been shown to be critical in maintaining graft patency after CABG. When the drug is given immediately after surgery, the one-year patency increases from 75 to 89%. In fact, it must be administered either orally or as a suppository, within the first 24 h, and perhaps the first 6 h after surgery, to demonstrate any benefit from its use. Trials have only proven a benefit from the administration of this drug for a period of one year. If the patient has had a previous MI, the drug should probably be continued indefinitely.

227 The major preoperative consideration is the patency of the airway. Upper mediastinal masses can result in occlusion of the trachea, especially after muscle tone has been blocked by paralytic agent. Initial evaluation includes assessing whether the patient can lie supine. Flow volume loops may reveal evidence of fixed extrinsic compression. If the patient has stridor and airway distress, management includes humidified oxygen, upright position, heliox (30% O_2, 70% helium) and early airway control.

Airway control in the OR is best assured in the nonparalysed patient. Intubation can be performed with a fibre-optic scope, or carefully 'breathing the patient down'. Rigid bronchoscopy should be available to intubate the airway should there be collapse of the trachea.

The majority of these lesions are not associated with tracheomalacia, but occasionally stenting is required postoperatively. Rarely, with tracheal invasion, tracheal resection may be required. Even more rarely, with major mediastinal masses, femoral cardiopulmonary bypass may be needed.

228 This represents a patient with an IABP placed for cardiogenic shock (**228**). There is an insufficient response. Discuss the aetiology.

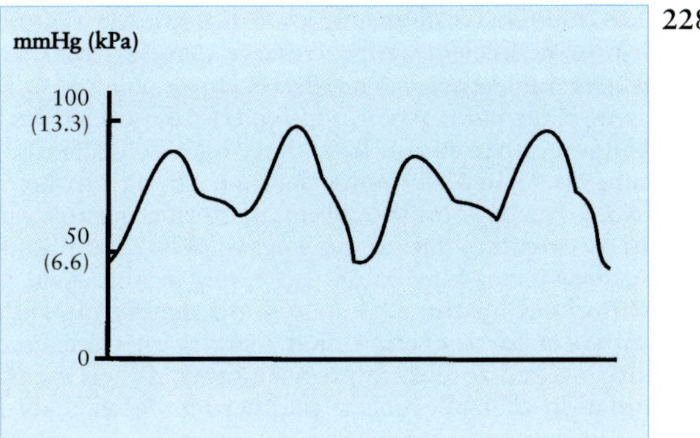

229 A patient develops persistent stridor following removal of a tracheostomy tube which has been in place for a month. In a stable patient what immediate diagnostic steps should be performed?

230 A chest radiograph obtained 4 h following tube thoracostomy (intercostal drainage) for pneumothorax is shown (**230**). The next step should be:
i. Placement of a second chest tube via the same incision.
ii. Placement of a second tube via a new incision.
iii. Pull the chest tube back 5 cm.
iv. Advance the chest tube 5 cm.
v. Increase suction from 20 cm of water to 25 cm of water.

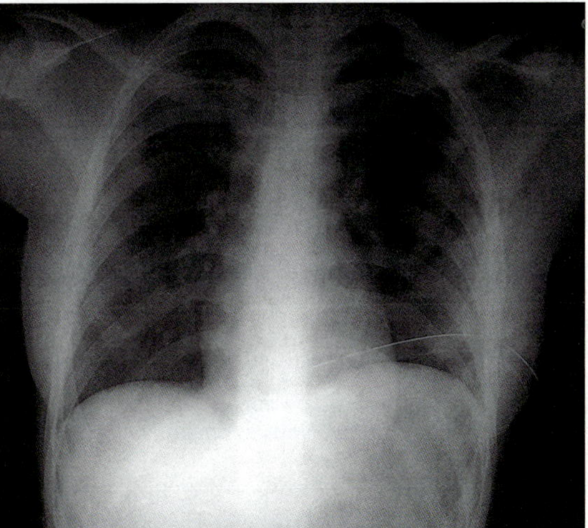

228 Ineffective augmentation can result for a number of reasons. A significant problem is insufficient cardiac reserve. A ventricular assist device may be required. Ineffective augmentation can also occur in children whose vessels are too pliable, as well as in older patients with extremely atherosclerotic and non-distensible vessels. If the balloon is placed too low, there may be decreased effectiveness. The most common cause is related to timing. Balloon timing can be made from an arterial pulse or an ECG. The balloon should inflate during diastole and can be triggered by the R wave so as to inflate during the T wave. A low amplitude R wave or rhythm disturbances such as atrial fibrillation can result in abnormal triggering. Arterial pressure trace, with good upstroke of at least 40 mmHg (5.3 kPa) can be used if the ECG is not sufficient for triggering or if there is interference due to cautery use. Wave-form is also needed to ensure proper timing. When measured through the balloon lumen, inflation should occur at the dicrotic notch. Late inflation, as shown in (**228**), will result in inadequate augmentation.

229 Plain PA and lateral chest radiographs with penetration may show an area of tracheal stenosis. Tracheal laminograms, if available, can show a continuous display of the stenotic area. CT or MRI give detailed information concerning the length and character of the stricture. Bronchoscopy should be part of the evaluation of tracheal stenosis. Flexible endoscopy visualizes the length and calibre of the stenosis and the health of the mucosa above and below the lesion. Measurements from the vocal cords and carina can be made to guide planned resection. Rigid bronchoscopy offers the additional element of dilatation which may obviate tracheostomy in critically compromised lumens. Laser resection of a short segment stenosis may give long-term patency, although many will recur. When surgical resection is anticipated, the exact anatomical location of the lesion is mandatory. Lesions in the upper two-thirds can usually be managed by a collar incision with or without a manubrial split. Lesions in the lower third of the trachea are generally approached through a right posterolateral thoracotomy (4th interspace). An armoured endotracheal tube and flexible bronchoscope should be available at the time of intubation. Sterile anaesthesia tubing to be placed over the drapes should be used when the distal trachea is intubated after resection of the stenotic segment. When the diseased area is mobilised, care should be taken to avoid disturbing the lateral entrance of the blood supply greater than 1 cm above and below the lesion. In most situations interrupted absorbable sutures should be used. Undue tension at the anastomosis can result in disruption. At the conclusion of the procedure, the chin should be anchored to the anterior chest wall with a heavy suture to prevent inadvertent extension of the neck. This can be removed within 5 days.

230 ii. The last hole of the chest tube is extrapleural. Avoiding this complication, of course, requires confirmation of intrapleural placement by feeling the lung tissue at the time of placement, advancing the tube to assure the proximal port is intrapleural, and by verifying respiratory fluctuation of the water column. A chest tube should never be advanced nor a new tube placed via a previously placed incision once the initial sterile prep has been broken.

231 What is the mechanism of action of ASA in patients with coronary artery disease?

232 Discuss indications and contraindications for closure of congenital VSDs.

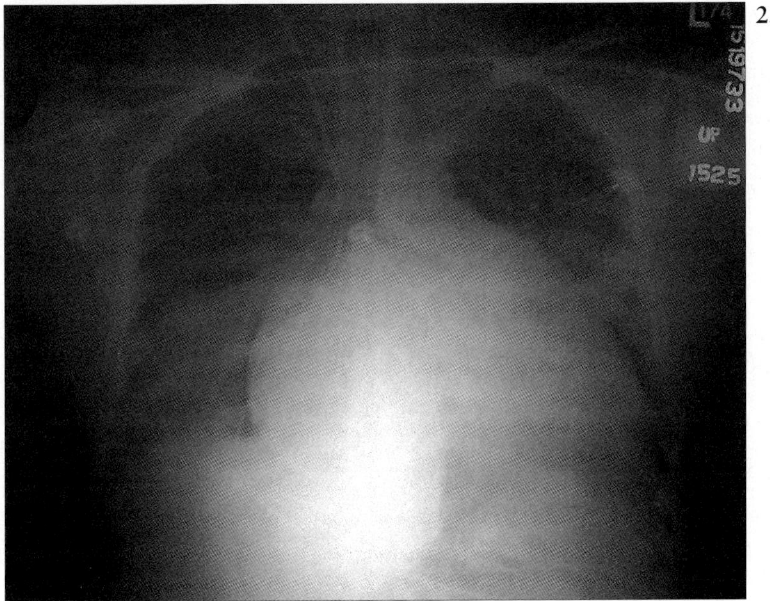

233

233 A patient with end stage heart disease is admitted to the CCU while awaiting heart transplant. There is extreme difficulty in obatining a wedge with a Swan catheter. This chest radiograph is obtained (**233**). What are your thoughts?

234 An 82-year-old woman presents with exertional syncope. Her exercise tolerance has declined over the past two years, such that she now has dyspnoea when climbing one flight of stairs. She has no cardiac risk factors. Echocardiography demonstrates a mean aortic valve gradient of 32 mmHg (4.3 kPa), a planimetrically determined valve area of 0.6 cm^2 and severe reduction of left ventricular function with concentric hypertrophy. Discuss the echocardiographic result, further diagnostic tests, prognosis and therapeutic options for this patient.

231 ASA functions as a platelet inhibitor by irreversibly inhibiting the cyclooxygenase enzyme within the platelet cytosol (see **226**). As a result of this, the formation of thromboxane A_2 from arachidonic acid (the latter derived from the platelet membrane) is blocked. As platelets lack nuclear material, there is no capacity to regenerate cyclooxygenase, and therefore the inhibition lasts for the duration of the platelet's survival. Other vascular cells, such as endothelial cells are inhibited by this drug; however, the enzymes can be synthesized *de novo* and prostacyclin production continues unabated. NSAIDs also inhibit platelet function by blocking cyclooxygenase; however, this inhibition is reversible and only lasts while the drug is in the circulation.

232 Indications for VSD closure include: juxta-arterial VSDs, especially if associated with aortic prolapse, inlet VSDs, uncontrolled CHF, failure to thrive, need for another cardiac procedure and/or recurrent respiratory problems. VSDs associated with high flow 'jets' are an increased risk for SBE. Large VSDs are characterized by having at least one of the following features: size >1/2 diameter of the aorta or >1 cm/m^2 BSA; Qp/Qs >2; pulmonary pressure/systemic pressure >0.5. These usually do not close spontaneously and it is recommended that they be operated on before two years of age to prevent progressive pulmonary vascular changes leading to irreversible pulmonary hypertension. Should there be minimal ('balanced') shunt, but not because the VSD is restrictive, there should be concern about pulmonary hypertension, or even flow reversal (Eisenmenger's syndrome). Fixed pulmonary hypertension >8 U/m^2 is a contraindication to closure.

233 Obviously, it will be difficult to 'float' a PAOC because of his dilated cardiomyopathy. The catheter is coiled in the right ventricle. Care should be taken when pulling it to avoid knotting.

234 This woman has severe aortic stenosis. Echocardiography is very accurate at identifying this if several types of determination are employed. Valve gradients may be determined by the continuity equation. A mean gradient over 50 mmHg (6.7 kPa) and a peak greater than 60 mmHg (8.0 kPa) are very suggestive of severe stenosis. Aortic valve area may be determined by Doppler (i.e. velocity) or planimetry (i.e. direct visualization of the valve orifice as well as aortic valve resistance (which is independent of gradient and flow)). All these results correlate strongly with gradients and areas determined by cardiac catheterization using the Gorlin formula. Catheterization is usually requested to assess coronary anatomy. Reduced LV function in this lady probably accounts for the relatively low measured gradient.

Symptomatic medical treatment of severe aortic stenosis in the elderly results in a two-year mortality rate of approximately 50%, about half of these from sudden death. Surgical treatment is associated with a mortality rate of about 3–5%, dependent on age, urgency, reoperation, LV function, coronary artery disease, atrial fibrillation and comorbidity. Survival following AVR is less than for the general population, being 75% at 5 years and 60% at 10 years (a distinct improvement over medical therapy). Percutaneous balloon aortic valvuloplasty has a high complication rate (25% (aortic regurgitation, cardiac rupture, stroke, MI, conduction abnormalities) and high recurrence rate (50–75% in 9 months) with a 30% mortality in 1 year. Its best indication may be in those patients who are not operative candidates, in whom it may improve function temporarily such that operation becomes possible.

235 Discuss the surgical management options in a patient who presents with increasing dyspnoea, a chest radiograph that suggests only left lung involvement and this CT scan (235). What are the indications for surgery in emphysema?

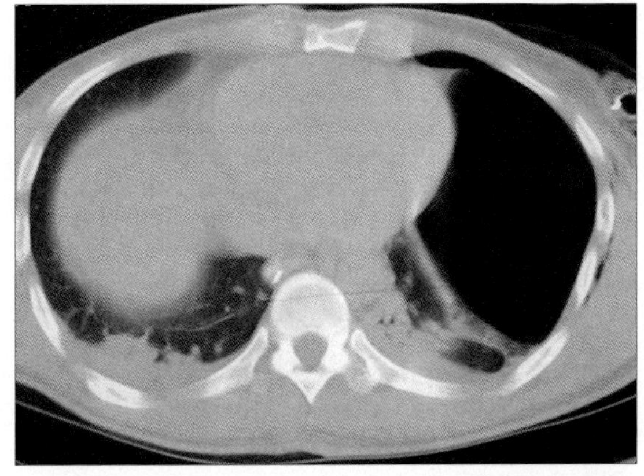

236 A 23-year-old man suffered a gun shot wound to the right groin. Two days following admission, he developed substernal chest pain. A chest radiograph is shown (236). Diagnostic options include which of the following?
i. Repeat chest radiograph, inspiration and expiration.
ii. Oesophageal swallows.
iii. ECG.
iv. Arterial blood gas.
v. Ventilation profusion scan.
vi. Cardiac catheterization.

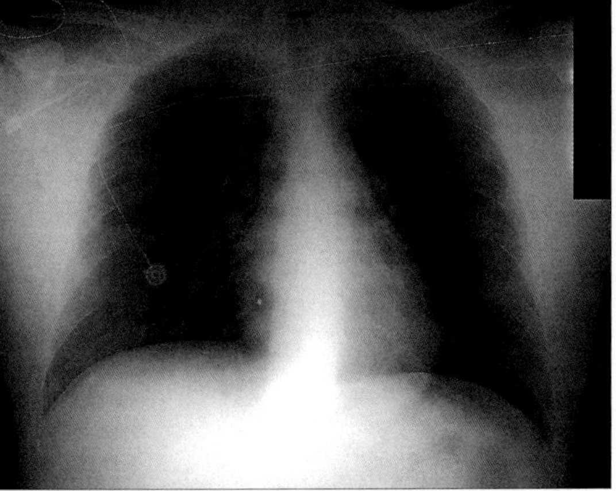

237 PFC may be seen in the term or near-term infant as a result of all the below except:
i. Meconium aspiration.
ii. Group B haemolytic streptococcal sepsis.
iii. Congenital diaphragmatic hernia.
iv. Congenital laryngotracheal oesophageal cleft.

235 Symptomatic bullae in patients without diffuse underlying emphysematous changes are usually apporached by thoracotomy and bullectomy or VATS (possibly with laser reduction).

Indications for surgery on patients with emphysema may include breathlessness, to improve chest wall function prior to transplantation, pneumothorax, bleeding, infection and cancer. The potential benefit depends upon the degree of compression of underlying normal lung. Ideally there should be the following:

- Bullae greater than 1/3–1/2 hemithorax.
- Normal underlying lung.
- None or easily controlled infection.
- FEV_1 greater than 0.8.
- No α-antitrypsin deficiency.

The patient here has predominately left upper lobe involvement, best approached by open bullectomy. There may be considerable normal lung tissue compressed by the bullae and lobectomy might remove a large amount of normal tissue.

236 iii, iv, v and **vi.** This patient has no evidence of pneumothorax. Oesophageal injuries are unlikely in a patient with a blast remote to the chest. Unless the patient has a pre-operative history suggesting oesophageal motility disorders, it is unlikely that the oesophagus is the source of the pain. If pulmonary embolization is considered, the appropriate first test is an ABG followed by VQ scan, if necessary. This patient had an abnormal ECG which revealed ischaemic changes; a cardiac catheterization confirmed the presence of bullet embolus to the coronary artery via a patent foramen of ovale. In general, the approach to this would be the same approach to any patient with coronary ischaemia. If there is a significant area of myocardium that is threatened, surgical removal and possible bypass might be required. Heparinization should be used. If the area of ischaemia is minimal, a nonoperative approach can be used. This patient underwent operative removal of embolism and had saphenous vein grafting.

237 iv. Persistent pulmonary hypertension or PFC may be seen in a variety of conditions. Meconium aspiration syndrome, beta-haemolytic streptococcal sepsis and congenital diaphragmatic hernia are classically associated with PFC. These were the first conditions treated with ECMO.

Congenital laryngotracheal oesophageal cleft is not associated with PFC unless there is an associated underlying cardiac or diaphragmatic defect.

There have been reports of repair of congenital LTE clefts using ECMO and allowing the repair to heal without subjecting the trachea to the barotrauma from conventional ventilation postoperatively.

238 This is a representation of the mitral valve, as it might be seen while performing mitral valve repair or replacement (**238**). The letters indicate structures that can be implicated in failure to come off bypass, ventricular rupture and/or poor ventricular function with decreased 10-year survival. What are they?

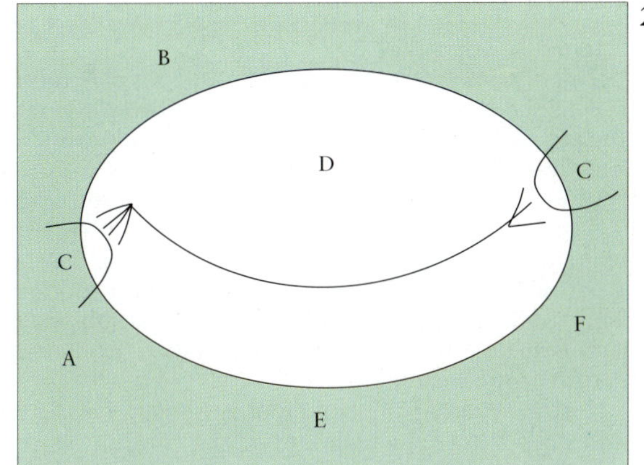

239 A 73-year-old patient, following bowel resection for adenocarcinoma of the colon, is hypoxic following the surgery. Her ventilator settings are FiO_2 50%, PEEP 5 cm H_2O, tidal volume is 750 ml, assist control rate of 12/min. Blood gases reveal a PO_2 of 65 mmHg (8.7 kPa), a PCO_2 of 45 mmHg (6.0 kPa), and a pH of 7.35 ([H⁺] 45). The chest radiograph obtained in recovery room is shown (**239**). The next step in the management is:

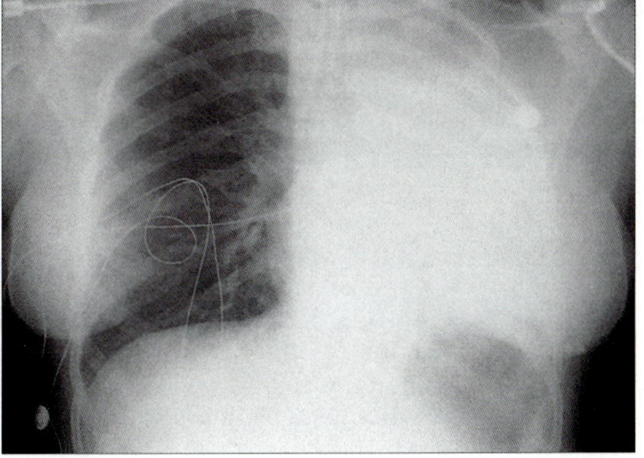

i. Increase the FiO_2 to 100%.
ii. Increase the PEEP to 7.5 cm H_2O.
iii. Increase the tidal volume to 1000 ml.
iv. Adjust the endotracheal tube.
v. Perform bronchoscopy.

240 A 70-year-old male patient who had recently had a colon resection, suffered a pulmonary embolus for which he was successfully treated with a pulmonary embolectomy. On the fourth postoperative day, the patient underwent a duplex scan of the leg veins which was normal. What further therapy is required?

238 A is the area of the circumflex artery. Sutures placed here may injure the vessel, leading to ischaemia.

B is area of the 'aortic curtain'. It is possible to injure the aortic valve here.

C is the papillary muscle-chord complex. It is felt that preserving either or both of the chordal attachments preserves ventricular function and results in better long-term function. The retention of the attachments may also reduce the risk of ventricular rupture. Additionally, excessive traction on the cords may lead to localized rupture.

D is the anterior leaflet. When performing mitral annuloplasty, some authors contend that if the posterior leaflet height is not 'shortened', it may 'bang' into the anterior leaflet resulting in systolic anterior motion of the anterior leaflet or 'SAM'. This results in left ventricular outflow tract obstruction.

E is the annulus. Rupture can occur if an oversized valve is placed or if excessive decalcification is required.

F is the area of the conduction system. This is fairly deep and an extremely wide and deep suture might injure it, resulting in heart block. It is an area that is often asked about in exams, however!

239 iv. Proper placement of an endotracheal tube is assessed by auscultation of both hemithoraces, observation of bilateral excursion, and in the adult ensuring that the insertion at the teeth is approximately 22 cm. Main stem (bronchial) intubation usually occurs in the right side and the management is to withdraw the endotracheal tube and re-assess breath sounds. A differential diagnosis of partial right-sided collapse might also include occlusion of an anomalous tracheal origin of right upper lobe bronchus.

240 It has been generally accepted that patients surviving pulmonary embolectomy should be anticoagulated with heparin and warfarin, the latter for around 6 months. Despite this therapy, embolus may recur and therefore some surgeons have recommended that caval filters should be inserted in these patients.

IVC interruption with a filter (Greenfield) is not without risk. Some researchers have suggested that the incidence of venous thrombosis with such a filter is up to 40%. In the light of this, filter use should be individualized. Notably, if the patient developed the pulmonary embolus while on therapeutic anticoagulation, or if follow-up radiological studies demonstrate persistent clot in the femoral or iliac veins or the IVC despite anticoagulation, some form of device should be inserted to prevent recurrence. In some instances, for example with this case, the entire clot has embolized and there is little or no risk of recurrence of the clot if the patient risk factors are removed. It should be recalled that pelvic veins are also a probable site of thrombosis following colon surgery and/or malignancy.

241 A 16-year-old female, having sustained a stab wound in the left precordium, presents with confusion, jugular venous distension, tachypnoea and muffled heart sounds. Her systolic blood pressure fluctuates, being intermittently heard at 95 mmHg (12.7 kPa) but more consistently at 80 mmHg (10.7 kPa). Large bore IVs have been started and fluid administered. Her chest radiograph is shown (**241**). The next step could include:

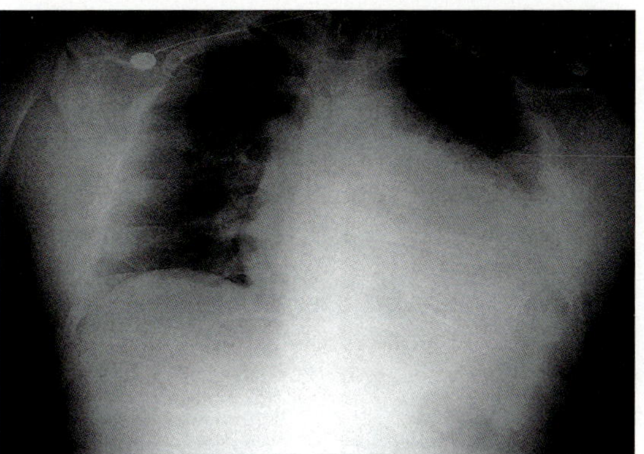

i. Pericardiocentesis.
ii. CT scan of the chest.
iii. Transthoracic echo.
iv. Observation.
v. Immediate intubation.

242 What medications could be used in coronary artery disease patients not tolerating ASA?

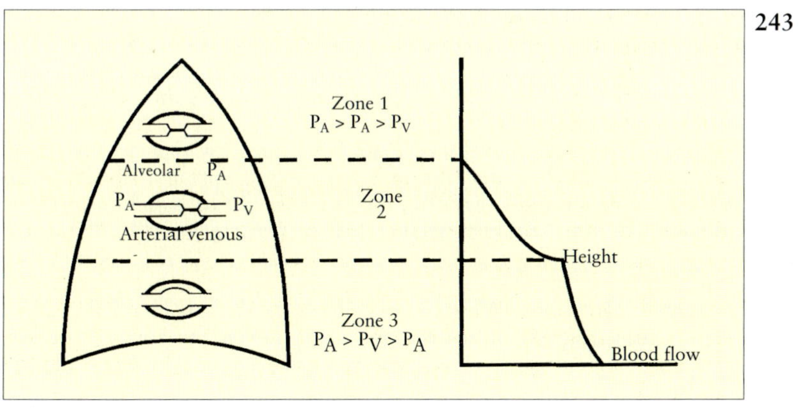

243 Ideally, a PAOC should lie in which of these 'zones'?

241 i. This patient has pericardial tamponade. Beck's triad of muffled heart sounds, pulsus paradoxus (>10 mmHg (1.3 kPa)) and jugular venous distension is present in only 10% of such cases. Without definite clinical signs, options include placement of measuring CVP, echo and/or pericardial window.

Transthoracic echo may not detect small injuries. If small fluid collections are noted, exploration should probably be performed. Transoesophageal echo is more accurate, but requires sedation and may not be practical. Liberal use of subxiphoid pericardial windows have a 70% negative exploration rate, but is useful in a patient undergoing laparotomy.

In a patient who clearly has pericardial tamponade, the best approach is to go staight to median sternotomy. Pericardiocentesis, with or without placement of an aspiration catheter, may be performed in selected circumstances prior to induction to avoid a cardiac decompensation. It must be stressed that pericardiocentesis is not definitive therapy. Blood may clot and the aspirate yield no result. The role of pericardiocentesis in penetrating trauma should be limited to those patients who appear acutely unstable and who will undergo surgical exploration regardless of the result. CT scan is not appropriate.

242 In patients in whom larger doses of ASA (325 mg/day) are not tolerated due to GI effects (e.g. dyspepsia, gastritis), consideration should be given to the use of smaller doses of ASA (e.g. 75 mg/day). Studies have demonstrated that this smaller dose is equally effective at increasing graft patency long term, and yet there is a significant decrease in the amount of GI bleeding which may occur.

Although many authors have suggested that the phosphodiesterase inhibitor dipyridamole should be used as an alternative drug, no prospective trial has demonstrated that it is effective in promoting graft patency. This probably relates to the difficulty in obtaining adequate serum levels of the drug with oral administration and therefore, this drug should not be recommended.

Trials have shown beneficial effects of postoperative administration of sulphinpyrazone as well as the anticoagulant warfarin in improving graft patency. Although equally effective as ASA, the use of these drugs may be associated with increased side effects including bleeding.

Triclopidine is a recently developed drug which acts by irreversibly blocking the interaction between platelets and fibrinogen at the glycoprotein IIb/IIIa receptor. At moderate doses (250 mg bid), this drug has been shown to maintain improved graft patency. Prominent side effects include a risk of neutropenia (4%) and a possible increase in alkaline phosphatase.

243 These are the so called 'West's zones'. In zone 1, there is no flow. In zone 2, there is obstruction downstream of the pulmonary artery. In zone 3, the vessels are open from pulmonary arterial to the venous side. Thus, a PAOC tip placed in this area will most accurately reflect left atrial pressure.

244 This patient was involved in a RTA (244). He suffered multiple pelvic, long bone and intracranial injuries. He developed ARDS and requires increasing ventilatory support, with subsequent cardiac compromise. What is the role of ECMO?

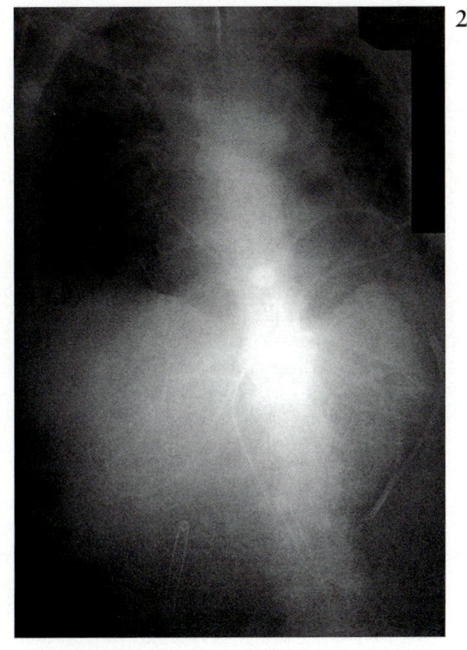

244

245 A male patient post-CABG is bleeding at a rate of 250 ml/h for 4 hours. There are no other sites of active bleeding. His coagulation parameters are as follows:

INR   1.7
Fibrinogen   1.1 g/l (110 mg/dl)
PTT   40 s
Platelets   95 (95 × 10⁹/l)
TT   17 s
Thromboelastogram (245)

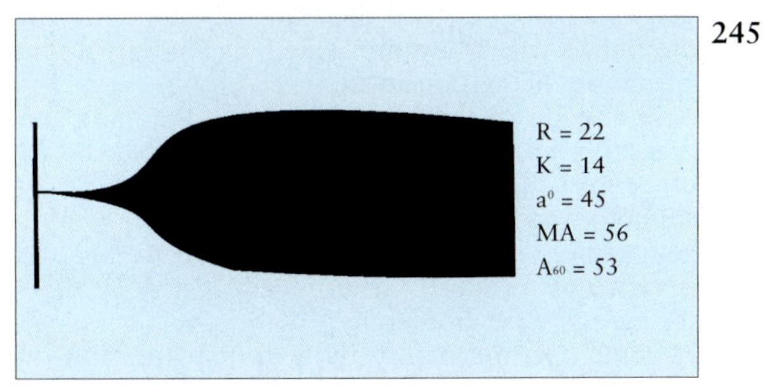

245

How should this patient be managed? Should blood products be given?

246 Discuss the physiological evaluation and surgical options in treating sympto-matic 'diffuse' emphysema.

244 The role of ECMO in trauma patients is still experimental. Groups that advocate it recommend early intervention, i.e. before >5 days of ventilation. One series reported 63% survival, with a 75% incidence of bleeding. The average duration was 12 days. In rare circumstances it may be considered, therefore, but if bleeding represents a major threat (e.g. with head injuries or spinal contusions) it should not be used.

245 Coagulation abnormalities after open heart surgery are relatively common as a result of haemodilution and consumption of platelets during exposure of the blood to the bypass circuit. However, coagulopathy as a primary cause of excessive bleeding after surgery is less common than bleeding due to inadequate surgical haemostasis. As a general rule, patients with bleeding >500 ml in any hour, or >250 ml for 4 h should be re-explored before giving blood products. After removal of the clot, sites of surgical bleeding can be ruled out. Only if there is persistent oozing with the sternum re-opened should blood products be considered. In general, due to the likelihood of platelet dysfunction after bypass, platelet concentrates should be the first product administered in that situation. The TEG is normal.

246 In more than 80% of emphysema cases, the risk/benefit of surgery is not clear because of associated diffuse emphysematous changes. Patients that appear to benefit most are 'pink puffers' as opposed to 'blue bloaters' who are characterized by significant hypoxia, CO_2 retention, recurrent infections, hypoventilation and heart failure. Physiological testing that suggests a possible benefit from resection includes finding that plethysmographic calculation of FRC is much greater than helium determination, implying that the bulla(e) is (are) trapping a large volume of gas. Evidence of parenchymal 'crowding' can also be obtained from inspiration/expiration radiographs, angiogram and dynamic CT scan. All these findings imply that eliminating the bullae will allow the remaining underlying lung to recover some of its normal 'elastic recoil' and function.

In the abscence of an obviously 'dominant' bullae, one surgical option is 'lung reduction surgery'. One method advances the role of VATS laser shrinkage. The other, in conjuction with an intense period of perioperative physiotherapy, utilizes sternotomy to resect bullae. Staple lines are reinforced with bovine pericardium. The goal of both is to preserve as much functioning tissue as possible. The best approach is yet to be absolutely determined. It may be that the benefit seen is primarily from the agressive physiotherapy.

Some patients require lung transplantation due to the onset of cor pulmonale and/or diffuse disease. One temporizing option, if there is a significant bulla, is external drainage with a catheter. The goal of this is to reduce O_2 requirements and allow rehabilitation of the chest wall for subsequent transplantation.

247 Match the drug with its haemodynamic effect:
i. Esmolol.
ii. Nitroprusside.
iii. Dobutamine.
iv. Adrenaline.

MAP	CO	SVR	PCWP
none/i	i	d	d
d	i or d	d	d
i	i	d	d
d	d	none	none

(i = increase; d = decrease)

248 A 45-year-old woman is unable to be weaned off CPB following mitral valve repair. The CI is 1.5 l/min/m², left atrial pressure is 10 mmHg (1.3 kPa), right atrial pressure is 25 mmHg (3.3 kPa) despite significant inotropic and vasodilator drugs including amrinone (aminophylline, milrinone), adrenaline and dobutamine and IABP support. Transoesophageal echocardiography shows an adequate mitral valve repair. The next course of action should be:
i. Addition of noradrenaline to the treatment regime.
ii. Maintenance of CPB for 2 h.
iii. Installation of a RV assist device.
iv. Installation of a LV assist device.
v. Installation of a biventricular assist device.

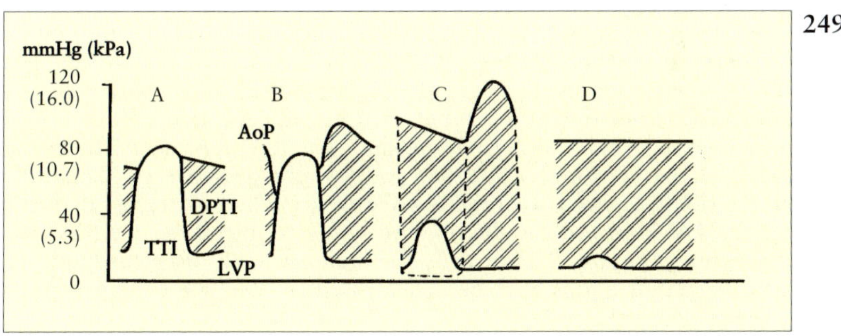

249 What is represented here (**249**)?

247 Esmolol is a short acting beta-blocker. It has been used to control supra-ventricular tachycardia and postoperative hypertension. Severe hypotension is the most common adverse reaction. Nitroprusside is both an arterial and venovaso-dilator. It is used as an antihypertensive agent. Dobutamine is a positive inotropic, chronotropic and vasodilating agent. It is used primarily to improve myocardial contractility and stroke volume. Adrenaline is a naturally occurring catecholamine which is a potent vasoconstrictor.

Drug	MAP	CO	SVR	PCWP	Heart rate
Esmolol	d	d	none	none	d
Nitroprusside	d	i[1]	d	d	i
Dobutamine	none/i[2]	i	d	d	i/none
Adrenaline	i	i	i[3]	i	i

[1] Occasionally decreases CO.
[2] Can decrease blood pressure if insufficient preload.
[3] At low doses can see slight vasodilatation with predominately inotropic effect.

248 iii. This patient has right ventricular failure as evidenced by a low CI and high right atrial pressures and normal left atrial pressures. This could be the result of a stunned myocardium and there is a fair chance of this recovering if the right ventricle is adequately supported by means of a RV assist device. Waiting too long on CPB could further damage her coagulation system and possibly lead to vital organ damage. In the absence of left heart failure a LV assist device or a biventricular device is not indicated.

249 These are the representations of myocardial supply and demand relationships. Greater than 80% of coronary flow, and hence subendocardial perfusion, occurs during diastole, from the beginning of isometric relaxation and the start of iso-volaemic contraction. This Diastole Pressure Time Index (DPTI) represents supply. Myocardial oxygen demands are reflected by the Tension Time Index (TTI), the period of contraction reflected by the LV pressure curve during systole. The ratio of DPTI/TTI represents supply/demand relationships. With tachycardia, for example, the duration of diastolic flow is increased, resulting in decreased DPTI.

Figure A represents the normal relationship. Figure B represents the effects of an IABP which increases 'supply' and has some slight decrease in 'demand' due to decreased afterload. Figure C represents a LV device which decreases demand due to emptying the LV, markedly reducing the work required, as well as increasing diastolic pressures. Figure D represents the state on CPB after cardioplegia, when myocardial oxygen demands have been decreased to 10–20% of that of the normal working heart.

250a 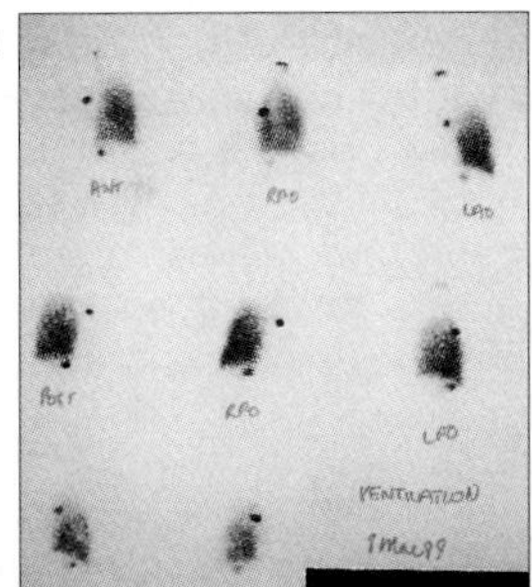

250b

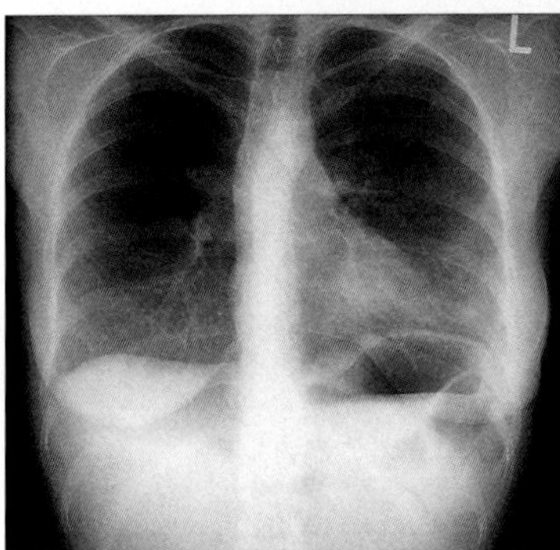

250c

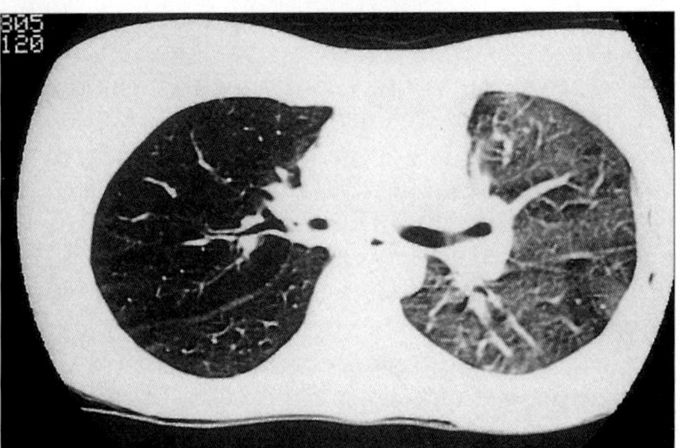

250d

250 A young woman presents with increasing stridor. She has a history of multiple blunt trauma two years previously. Review of her hospital course revealed that she had required prolonged ventilator support for presumed pulmonary contusion. It is also noted that for a period of time, she had a documented pneumothorax, which persisted despite tube thoracostomy. No airleak was noted and the pneumothorax gradually resolved spontaneously. A ventilation perfusion scan, CT scan and bronchogram are presented (**250a–d**). Bronchoscopy confirms the injury. She should undergo:
i. Observation.
ii. Stenting.
iii. Pneumonectomy.
iv. Sleeve resection of the right mainstem.

251 A 45-year-old male with injuries sustained in a RTA presents to the emergency room comatose with a systolic arterial blood pressure of 90 mmHg (12.0 kPa), a heart rate of 110 b.p.m., and a respiratory rate of 33 breaths/min. Soon after intubation and ventilation, he deteriorates. You:
i. Immediately open the chest and perform open cardiac massage.
ii. Transfuse blood.
iii. Auscultate the chest.
iv. Do a diagnostic peritoneal lavage.
v. Reintubate the patient.

250 This patient suffered a traumatic disruption of the right mainstem bronchus which healed with resultant stricture. Tracheo-bronchial injuries following blunt trauma occur within 2 cm of the carina in 80% of cases. A persistent pneumothorax without airleak suggests total transection with mediastinal tissues occluding the bronchus. When diagnosed late, sleeve resection and reconstruction is preferred if there has been no intervening pulmonary sepsis resulting in gross parenchymal destruction. Usually, the hypoxic pulmonary response will resolve over time, as occurred in this patient.

251 iii. There are multiple causes for arrest in the trauma patient after intubation and beginning of ventilation. These causes for arrest include endotracheal tube malposition, increased intrathoracic pressure and metabolic problems. During intubation, visualization of the endotracheal tube passing through the cords is imperative for correct placement of the endotracheal tube. Auscultation of the chest for breath sounds with ventilation and listening over the stomach for air entry during bagging are helpful. Since in the trauma situation it is not always possible to visualize the vocal cords, some people have advocated the addition of a CO_2 sensor to the endotracheal tube. If no CO_2 is being produced, the endotracheal tube is in the wrong position. With the initiation of ventilation, rapid increases in the intrathoracic pressure may decrease venous return to the heart, thus precipitating cardiac arrest in the trauma patient with an intravascular volume deficit. Additionally, increased intrathoracic pressure with ventilation increases the size of a pneumothorax and produces a tension pneumothorax, which should be detected by auscultation and percussion. Patients with blunt chest trauma and a closed pneumothorax are at risk. Needle aspiration and placement of a chest tube will rapidly reverse an arrest secondary to a tension pneumothorax.

In the trauma situation, it is not unusual to have either penetrating injuries or blunt injuries with an opening from the bronchus into the vascular circulation. Aggressive ventilation may lead to air passage into the circulation which creates an air lock in the outflow tract. This may be treated by placing the patient in the left chest up, head down position. If the patient is haemodynamically unstable, this may be impossible. Advancing a central line into the right ventricle and aspirating may eliminate air in the right ventricular outflow tract. Open cardiac massage, aspiration of the ventricle, aspiration of air from the coronary arteries have all been used to treat this condition. In addition, hyperbaric oxygenation may be of some use in the stable patient. This has been more frequently used for neurological compromise related to air embolization. Finally, hyperventilation itself creates abnormalities in CO_2 and calcium metabolism which may precipitate an immediate arrest. Hypocarbia can result in systemic vasodilatation (although it paradoxically leads to cerebrovascular vasoconstriction) and the acute respiratory alkalosis can cause an acute decrease in the concentration of ionized calcium.

252 Analyse the right atrial and pulmonary waveforms (252a–c).

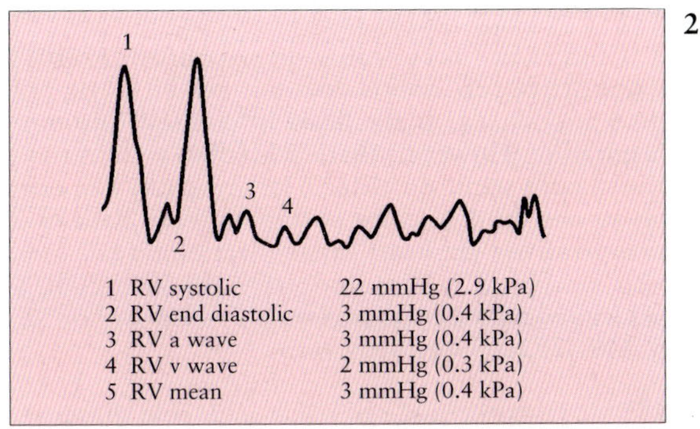

252a

1	RV systolic	22 mmHg (2.9 kPa)
2	RV end diastolic	3 mmHg (0.4 kPa)
3	RV a wave	3 mmHg (0.4 kPa)
4	RV v wave	2 mmHg (0.3 kPa)
5	RV mean	3 mmHg (0.4 kPa)

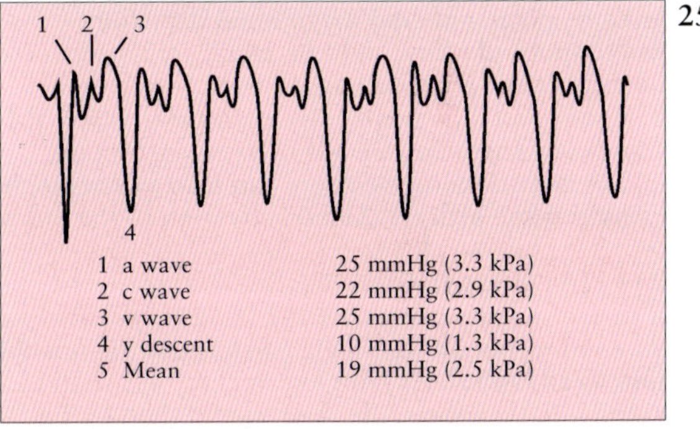

252b

1	a wave	25 mmHg (3.3 kPa)
2	c wave	22 mmHg (2.9 kPa)
3	v wave	25 mmHg (3.3 kPa)
4	y descent	10 mmHg (1.3 kPa)
5	Mean	19 mmHg (2.5 kPa)

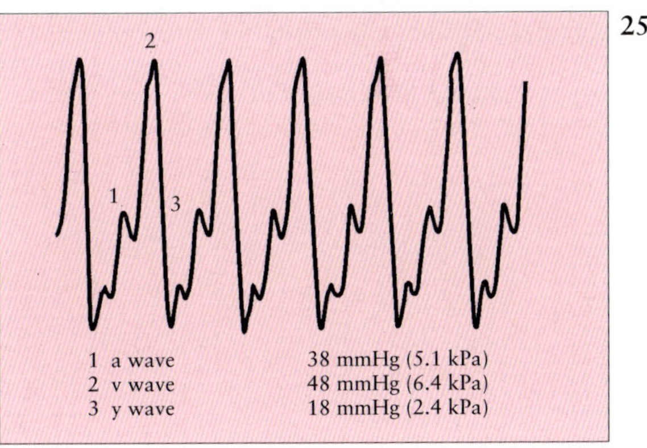

252c

1	a wave	38 mmHg (5.1 kPa)
2	v wave	48 mmHg (6.4 kPa)
3	y wave	18 mmHg (2.4 kPa)

253 List potential impacts that CPB can have on renal function.

254 A 60-year-old female, four weeks after cerebral contusion, develops acute chest pain, hypotension (systolic blood pressure 80 mmHg (10.7 kPa)), dyspnoea and ECG changes of RBBB. Discuss the diagnosis and management of this patient.

252 1. Normal (**252a**).
2. Constrictive pericarditis or myopathy (**252b**). Note the predominant y descent. Constrictive pericarditis does not exhibit as significant a change in pulse pressure as does tamponade, as the heart is 'encased' and not so sensitive to changes caused by inspiration. However, there is a fall in right atrial pressure with inspiration (positive Kussmaul's sign). An element of myopathy can exist, resulting in low CO syndrome in up to one-third of cases postoperatively. Risk of death following resection is 5% if preoperative right heart catheterization reveals pressure >16 mmHg (2.1 kPa), 10% if >20 mmHg (2.7 kPa) and 30% if >30 mmHg (4.0 kPa). Cardiac tamponade is associated with a predominant x descent without a significant y descent.
3. MR (**252c**). Note the v wave.

253 1. Hypothermia can result in a 'cold diuresis', related in part to decreased cortical blood flow. This is counterbalanced by haemodilution, but can lead to excessive volume, potassium and magnesium depletion.
2. Nonpulsatile flow may be associated with increased vasoconstriction and subsequently occult renal damage.
3. Renin and aldosterone are increased, which favours sodium retention and potassium loss. Angiotensin leads to vasoconstriction.
4. Trauma to blood elements can lead to haemoglobinuria, platelet plugging and increased tissue oedema due to activation of the inflammatory cascade.

254 The presentation suggests a significant pulmonary embolism (PE). Initial support includes administering oxygen, possibly intubation, and if hypotension persists, inotropes as well as heparinization. If possible, diagnosis can be confirmed by lung scan, spiral CT, angiogram, or occasionally by transoesophageal echocardiography. Lytic agents, the 'best' initial therapy for severe pulmonary embolism, would be relatively contraindicated due to the recent head injury. Closed pulmonary embolectomy might be tried, but with significant pulmonary embolism and persistent hypotension open embolectomy (despite the requirement for cardiopulmonary bypass) should be considered early. Earlier embolectomy results in improved outcomes, as delay often results in cardiac arrest with subsequent severe CNS injury.

255 A 57-year-old man is noted to have unifocal premature ventricular contractions, approximately 5/min, 3 h following completion of an uneventful four vessel bypass. The next step in management is:
i. Lidocaine bolus 100 mg.
ii. Start lidocaine (lignocaine) drip at 2 mg/min.
iii. Observation.
iv. Give 2 g of magnesium sulphate over 20 min.
v. Give K^+ and Mg^{2+} after checking serum concentrations.

256 A 35-year-old man sustained the cervical injury shown (**256**). Discuss the possible role of diaphragmatic pacing.

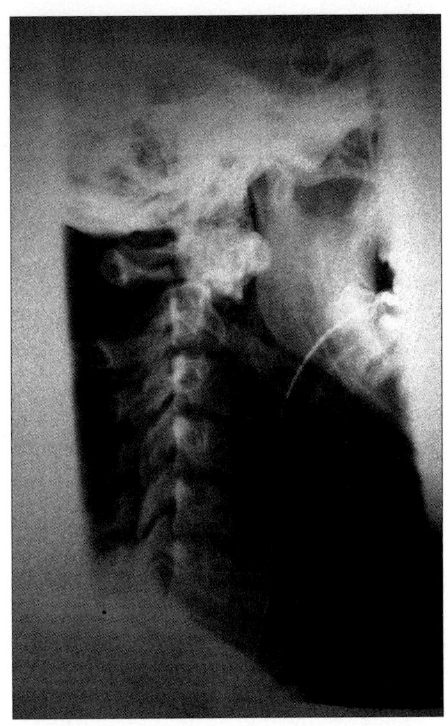

256

257 What options are available for patients in whom heparin cannot be used for running the cardiac bypass circuit?

255 Following cardiac surgery, VTs occur in up to 30% of patients. The significance of these arrhythmias is not entirely clear. The majority of postoperative VTs are both benign and transient and, other than correcting electrolyte abnormalities or other inciting causes, do not require specific treatment or monitoring. Issues related to the benefit of antidysrhythmic agents are confounded by their association with complications, including negative inotropism and proarrhythmia rates of up to 15%. There does not appear to be a clear-cut benefit of routine prophylaxis against arrhythmias, particularly VTs, except for specific situations.

Postoperative VTs are related to hypomagnesaemia and hypokalaemia. Hypomagnesaemia occurs in up to 70% of patients post pump. Inciting factors include preoperative use of diuretics, digoxin and beta-blockers, diabetes, intra-operative dilution, and postoperative loss of magnesium as a consequence of hypothermia and pump-induced diuresis. It should be noted that supplementation, regardless of the serum levels, has been shown to reduce the incidence and severity of VTs following myocardial infarction and cardiac surgery.

Indications for antidysrhythmics have traditionally included multiple (>6/min) PVCs, R-on-T phenomenon, multifocal PVCs or more complex rhythms including bigeminy or ventricular tachycardia. Many centres currently treat PVCs >10/min only if they persist despite magnesium and potassium supplementation. Transient ventricular tachycardia, bigeminy or trigeminy without hypotension may be managed in a similar fashion.

256 Diaphragmatic pacing may be indicated in patients suffering from idiopathic central alveolar hypoventilation, organic brain stem lesions, lesions of the cervical chord, some neuromuscular disorders and possibly severe COPD. It is contraindicated if there is not a viable phrenic nerve, if there exists a severe chest wall deformity, and if the primary problem is weakness of the diaphragmatic musculature. All patients should have a tracheostomy. Possible benefits include increased freedom from ventilators and better quality of life. Leads are usually placed transthoracically, as in up to 75% of cases the C5 root joins the phrenic nerve in the thorax.

257 In a patient with a history of thrombocytopenia associated with heparin, there are several options available for the anticoagulation required for CPB including:

- Ancrod: this enzyme, derived from the Malayan Pit Viper, produces complete anticoagulation by defibrinogenation.
- Prostacyclin analogue (Iloprost): this drug has proven successful in preventing platelet thrombi formation during CPB; however, its systemic effects result in hazardous systemic hypotension.
- Low molecular weight heparins: these drugs have been successfully used in patients with this disease. Unfortunately, these heparins are not completely reversed by protamine, thus resulting in excessive postoperative bleeding in some patients.

258 What do the following volumes represent?

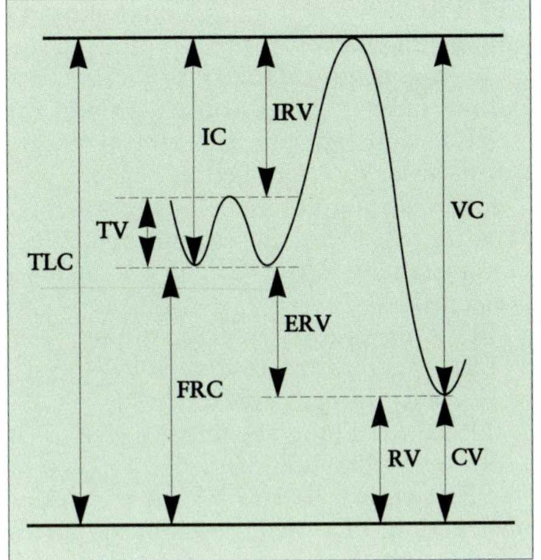

259 A 70-year-old woman, nine months following resection of a thoraco-abdominal aneurysm, presents with haematemesis and shock. After volume resuscitation restores vital signs, an endoscopy is performed which reveals a haemorrhagic lesion on the oesophageal wall at about 25 cm. The patient continues to be stable, and an aortogram is obtained (**259**). Discuss the management of this lesion.

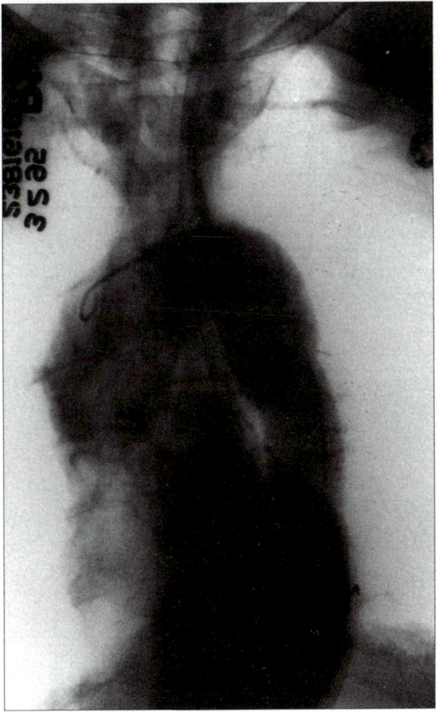

258 FRC = Functional residual capacity. It represents the volume of air left in the lung at the end of normal expiration and can be measured by gas washout or body plethysmography. Disparate values between the two methods indicates significant bullous disease, airway obstruction or other causes of poorly ventilated lung.

VC = vital capacity. If performed rapidly this is the FVC. In the presence of airway obstruction, FVC can be low.

CV = closing volume. This represents the volume at which airway closure occurs. It is increased in the supine position, with smoking and with age. Under ideal circumstances, RV = CV. If CV increases relative other voumes, there is increased atelactasis.

IRV = inspiratory reserve volume.

ERV = expiratory reserve volume.

IC = inspiratory capacity.

TLC = total lung capacity.

RV = residual volume.

FEV_1 refers to the volume exhaled in the first second. If there is airway obstruction, FEV_1 will be reduced, particularly as a ratio of FVC. FEV_1 occurs in the effort-dependent portion of expiration. FEF_{25-75} occurs in the effort-independent portion of expiration and is considered a useful test of small airway disease.

MVV, the maximum voluntary ventilation is particularly useful in determining risk of pulmonary surgery. Patients with less than 50% expected values have increased mortality and morbidity.

259 The suspicion of an aortoesophageal fistula becomes almost a certainty with a arteriogram demonstrating the graft-aortic anastomosis at the same level as the oesophageal 'lesion'. The patient should be explored through a left thoracotomy. If no or minimal contamination is encountered, then the vascular anastomosis should be resected and replaced with a new synthetic graft. If the contamination is substantial, then the problem becomes much more difficult. The involved aorta and graft should be extensively debrided to healthy tissue, the aortic stump should be securely closed and an extra-anatomic bypass from the ascending or transverse aorta to the aorta below the diaphragm should be constructed if possible. The oesophageal defect should be debrided and in the case presented it should be possible to primarily close it. The defect should then be reinforced with healthy tissue (pleural flap or old aneurysm wall) which would then be interposed between the oesophagus and the repaired aorta.

260 A 32-year-old immuno-compromised woman developed a pneumonic infiltrate complicated by haemoptysis. Sputum culture failed to define the aetiology. Bronchoscopy documented atypical acid-fast bacteria resistant to conventional antituberculous medication. The accompanying radiograph was taken after three months of antituberculous treatment (260). What treatment options are available?

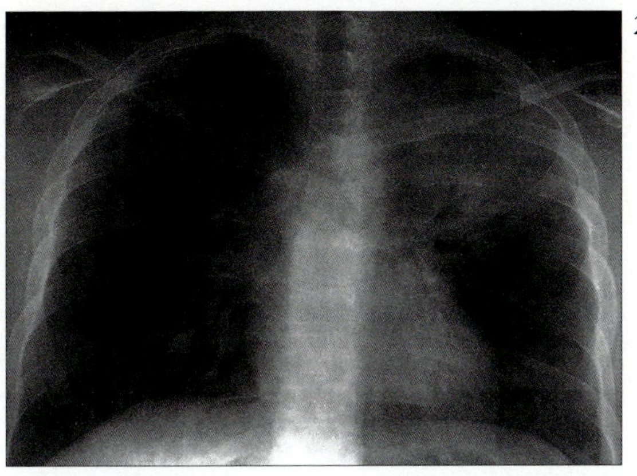

261 Discuss thrombocytopenia associated with heparin use.

262 A 55-year-old man presents with an acute anterior MI and receives tPA in the emergency room. Despite this, he rapidly deteriorates haemo-dynamically with a systolic blood pressure of 80 mmHg (10.7 kPa) requiring dopamine. He undergoes emergency cardiac catheterization which reveals an 80% left main stenosis. After it has been decided that this patient will require surgery his coagulation parameters are as follows:

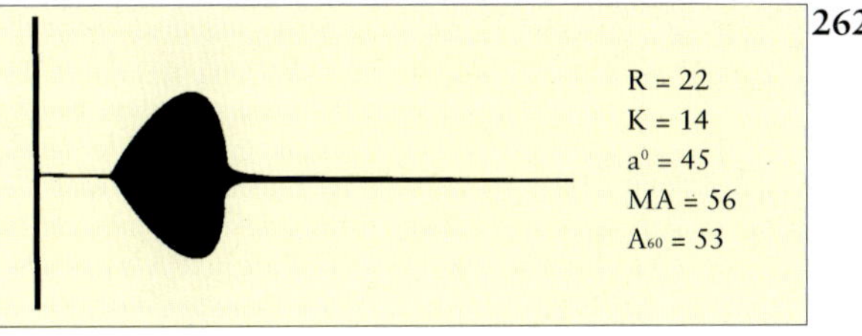

aPTT	60 s
PT	16 s
INR	1.4
Fibrinogen	0.7 g/l (70 mg/dl)
Platelets	175,000 (17.5 × 10⁹/l)

Discuss the use of blood products perioperatively.

260 The surgical management of pulmonary TB is usually reserved for failures of medical therapy or pulmonary structural complications. These include persistent positive sputum despite definitive antituberculous treatment, massive haemoptysis usually from a cavity colonized by *Aspergillus*, tuberculous empyema, bronchopleural fistula and inability to distinguish a pulmonary tuberculous lesion from malignancy. Tuberculous empyemas can be usually drained by a chest tube; if the underlying lung is entrapped, a decortication may be necessary. Associated bronchopleural fistulas may require lung resection or muscle flap closure. Complicated cavities and destroyed lung usually require pulmonary resection either by lobectomy or pneumonectomy.

261 Thrombocytopenia associated with heparin use is relatively common, seen in approximately 3–10% of individuals, occurring usually 6–12 days after initiation of therapy. This complication appears more frequently after exposure to bovine heparin than after porcine. Further, recent reports have demonstrated that the incidence after the use of low molecular weight heparin is significantly decreased as compared to the incidence with unfractionated heparin.

The mechanism by which the platelets are affected by heparin relates to antibodies directed to the Fc binding receptor on the platelet surface. This in turn may result in platelet activation. In fact, a proportion of patients with this complication subsequently progress to develop spontaneous thrombosis of venous and arterial vessels (heparin-associated thrombocytopenia and thrombosis, HATT).

This disease may be diagnosed by demonstrating the release of ADP or radiolabelled serotonin from pooled platelets after exposure to the test serum.

262 Fibrinolytics such as tPA and streptokinase have proven to be effective in decreasing the mortality of patients with acute MI, when the drugs have been administered early enough. Although tPA appears to be 'clot specific' *in vitro*, it still causes significant systemic fibrinogenolysis resulting in a drop in the functional fibrinogen level. Another consequence of this medication is platelet dysfunction. This probably results from cleavage of critical surface glycoproteins from the platelet membrane surface by plasmin, preventing the platelet from adhering to surfaces at sites of vascular injury.

As a result of these abnormalities, patients undergoing emergency open heart surgery will require liberal administration of blood products perioperatively. Cryoprecipitate should be given to replace the depleted fibrinogen and platelet concentrates should be ordered; however, both of these products should only be given after the completion of bypass just prior to the administration of protamine. Giving them earlier would lead to damage of the administered platelets by the bypass circuit and further consumption of the fibrinogen.

Index